Walking

The Beauty and Grace of Tightrope
Walking

*(Walking in the Mystery, the Power and the
Victory of the Cross)*

Raphael Bailey

Published By **Simon Dough**

Raphael Bailey

Walking: The Beauty and Grace of Tightrope Walking (Walking in the Mystery, the Power and the Victory of the Cross)

ISBN 978-1-998038-14-5

No part of this guidebook shall be reproduced in any form without permission in writing from the publisher except in the case of brief quotations embodied in critical articles or reviews.

Legal & Disclaimer

The information contained in this book is not designed to replace or take the place of any form of medicine or professional medical advice. The information in this book has been provided for educational & entertainment purposes only.

The information contained in this book has been compiled from sources deemed reliable, and it is accurate to the best of the Author's knowledge; however, the Author cannot guarantee its accuracy and validity and cannot be held liable for any errors or omissions. Changes are periodically made to this book. You must consult your doctor or get professional medical advice before using any of the suggested remedies, techniques, or information in this book.

Table Of Contents

Chapter 1: Walk Journal

Monday Morning Body Weight (in kilograms)

Day Time Started

Distance Covered Remarks Remark Monday

Tuesday

Wednesday

Thursday

Friday

Saturday

Sunday

Your walk journal should be a carefully organized and meticulous record of every day's walk. Not only will it benefit you in the short term, but it has additional long-term advantages as well. Make sure to create one today! The minimum time for active walking should be twenty minutes; thirty minutes is ideal. Those with health issues must get approval from their doctor before beginning to plan walks; however, walking is much simpler medically than other forms of exercise.

One more set of important details to keep track of during these eight weeks: your Nutrition Journal. While it will require more time and effort than keeping a walk journal, consider it as an investment for long term success.

Nutrition Journal: Day 1

Meal Time Food Item Units Pre-walk Post-walk Breakfast Lunch Snacks Evening Dinner

Sir Isaac Newton famously noted in his laws of motion that bodies tend to remain in an equilibrium state. These same laws hold true in the world of psychology as well, where one must first break through inertia to achieve progress. If you are just starting out and don't have that inertia to break through, consider yourself fortunate and take your first steps. On the other hand, if it does exist, don't despair; knowledge is power - and in this case it comes in its strongest form: awareness of your own weak point. From here, you can only progress. Even though the obstacle is familiar to you, don't underestimate its power. Make the most of each day's walk by visualizing its successful conclusion and staying positive throughout it all. Positivity is essential, so keep away from those with negative vibes to maximize your progress on your walk and overall wellness. Declare your intention of taking the eight weeks walk challenge in front of those closest to you: spouse, children, relatives and friends - anyone who loves you and will support you either directly by joining you as a walk buddy or indirectly by raising your morale.

For your walk, you will need some essential items: comfortable socks and shoes, sensible clothing, and a device that displays time. DVD players, IPods, headphones etc.

are not necessary but often help speed up the process for many. For this program, I ask you to keep it simple and close to the essentials. Avoid carrying any devices other than a watch. In humid or hot weather, make sure you bring plain water with you for hydration - this helps avoid dehydration. For a half an hour walk, there's no need to add salts or anything else to the water you carry. In colder climates, cover your head and ears properly with warm clothes before heading out for your walk. If you choose evening as your time for walking, make sure it is well lit and safe beforehand. Initially, we will walk for thirty continuous minutes at a pace comfortable for us during these first few weeks.

Walking, like other exercises, should be broken up into three phases: warm up; the activity (such as running or playing football or cricket); and cool down. Walking itself can serve as either a warm up or cool down for other exercises too - how does one go about warming up and cooling down for a walk? It's simple! Maintaining the intensity of our warm up and cool down walks slightly lower than that of the main walk will achieve optimal results. Five minutes should be allocated for each warm up walk, followed by five minutes for cooling down. Thus, a thirty minute walk will actually take thirty minutes to complete. At fifteen minutes into the journey, you will reach midway point. If the circuit chosen for a walk is noncircular and allows for mathematical calculations, one may walk for fifteen minutes from their starting point and then return, warming up in the first five minutes and cooling down in the last five.

Before you begin walking, it is important to know that most walkers require food in their stomach and enough calories stored for sustained energy levels. This information is especially pertinent for those who choose to walk first thing in the morning, right after they have woken up. They should consume a light breakfast and also some fluids like water or fruit juice before setting off on their walk. Give your body complex carbohydrates that take some time to digest and are released gradually. A banana or two medium sized toasts will always be more beneficial than glucose or fructose that's absorbed immediately after ingestion. There is a delicate balance to be struck when taking pre-walk meals. Only those who eat regularly know the difference between a stomach that's filled enough for walking and one that's too full. You must remember this distinction and plan your early morning walks accordingly. Additionally, no matter when or how often you decide to walk, never start off on an empty stomach nor overfill it.

One more fundamental human physiological function should be remembered: breathing deeply and efficiently. Children breathe naturally and efficiently at all times. For changing the pressure over their lungs, people use a diaphragm: a membrane that separates the cavity in which their lungs reside from that in which stomach and other internal organs reside. At any given moment, they can take in all the oxygen their bodies require and push out any deoxygenated air from their system. Unfortunately, many adults tend to forget this good practice and start breathing from their chest with less involvement of the diaphragm. As a walker, it is in your best interests to learn how to breathe from the diaphragm. It is so effortless that once you become conscious of doing this, your body will gradually begin shifting towards breathing in this manner throughout all situations - not just while walking. Start by placing your hand over your belly. Inhale and build pressure within your abdominal cavity so that your hand rises with air filled in it. Squeeze inward to exhale, as your hand moves inward. Practice it with and without hands until you learn to control your breathing in the abdominal cavity. This is a form of yoga practice known as hathyoga and the various pranayaams are done there as the science of life control through breathing. The breathing prescribed there is diaphragmatic, while in kapaal bhaati it's exaggerated.

Week 1

For the first week, our primary concerns should be time and consistency. There's no need to worry about speed, intensity or distance covered in thirty minutes; simply walk for thirty minutes every other day without stopping. For this initial week we will avoid uphill walks or those on uneven or unpaved surfaces in order to minimize obstacles and keep things simple.

Success, even small victories, are essential in building and maintaining motivation. That is why it is important to plan your walk ahead of time and stick with it; without maps you won't know the route as accurately as possible. Parks typically feature walking/jogging tracks, streets usually feature sidewalks, playgrounds usually feature either marked or unmarked perimeter tracks for running or walking on. Your choice is important as once it clicks you will feel more energised while out on your walk and may come in handy on those challenging days!

Are you mentally prepared and committed for the circuit? Have you planned out every detail in your head? Have taken enough calories before leaving and are dressed and ready to go. Congratulations on taking that first step on your path towards holistic fitness - I wish you luck and success, though I cannot take that first step anymore, except through vicariously. But at least now I get to accompany you every day as we move towards our goals together!

Start slowly; the first five minutes should be for warming up. Take deep breaths from your diaphragm and focus upon breathing deeply from your diaphragm. Turn on some music if you have it or run that track of positive thoughts through your mind to keep yourself focused upon yourself and the goal. Keep your lateral vision sharp when walking on sidewalks or crossing rough patches on the ground; alertness helps avoid injuries and accidents and contributes to success in a complementary manner. Don't rush at first - remember the basic idea is to enjoy yourself while completing this circuit successfully!

Establish and understand your normal stride. A brief digression on stride length is acceptable here; it was once believed that by elongating one's stride one could walk faster. Now it is known that it's not the length of paces but rather how many paces per minute matter when walking. So, walk naturally, letting your arms swing freely without trying to control their movement; their progress will be closely observed in later weeks.

After having completed five minutes of walking, you are now ready to set your pace for the next twenty minutes. If you feel that continuing with the pace from your warm-up walk on this first day will benefit you more, do so without feeling any pressure or need for conformity. It's completely up to you - there is no pressure or expectation here! Your program, your day and your rules should always remain unchanged: in order to form a habit an activity must be repeated with pleasure. Our plan is that walking will bring us joy every day so that it becomes an enjoyable habit that becomes second nature. So enjoy every step of the journey! Enjoy your favorite song, sing aloud if you feel inspired, or simply listen and take in the atmosphere without any mechanical devices other than a watch to keep time. Don't get bogged down with those earphones; leave them at home. Your senses should remain open to everything around you - keep your mobile on silent mode if possible and turn off notifications altogether if possible. No need for fancy devices that track every second your pulse rate, blood pressure and oxygen consumption. A walk is only half physical; the other half mental and spiritual. It helps you connect with yourself - similar to meditation - while connecting you to the world outside. We'll explore more of this in the seventh week.

Pay attention to your body's response during this activity. Perspiration is a sign of healthy metabolism when faced with increased exertion. Heavy sweating should serve as a reminder that it's time to replenish fluids. Don't worry if your heart starts beating faster at some point during the walk; that is completely normal and expected! There may be some heaviness in your shins which could later develop into mild pain when squatting. This condition, known as shin splint, occurs due to unbalanced muscular development above your ankles. Once your body adjusts and the muscles develop properly, any pain should vanish. To help muscles grow and develop, combine stretching exercises with simple exercises. However, if there's anything unsettling, stop immediately, inspect it, and determine whether it's serious or mild. If it is severe, discontinue the walk and consult your doctor; if not, continue walking as normal. Don't forget to slow your pace down in the last five minutes by walking at a slower pace than your main twenty minute walk. After arriving home, take a shower, have breakfast and then head off for work. When leaving or returning to your workplace, you may only get a momentary break for dry-off and a quick bite before beginning or continuing work. Try to incorporate this all seamlessly and unobtrusively into your routine so it becomes an easily integrated part of it.

Routine for Week One:

Chapter 2: Monday Through Saturday: Walk 30 Minutes

Rest 15 Minutes

Rest an additional 15 minutes before continuing your walk. Rest again for 30 seconds then walk for 30 more minutes, taking breaks to rest as needed. For each of the seven days following Week 1, aim to complete 30 minutes of physical activity each day, ending each session with 30 minutes of walking resting between each one.

On day three of the first week, which is Monday morning, there will be an adjustment period. On your second walk of the week, you may choose to follow a similar pattern as on day one or make it more interesting by altering your route or increasing your walking speed every alternate round or minute depending on whether you are taking rounds around a garden pathway, playground or walking on an extended circuit. For your next two walk days, keep it casual. Remember that this first week is for becoming familiar with and enjoying the activity - there's no need to rush. If you don't want any changes made, leave everything as-is on day one. Finally, remember to record every detail of your walk in your journal each day. In the "Remarks" column, you can record any physiological, physical or mental insights you may have gained during this eight week period, such as increased appetite, general fatigue, muscle aches, positive moods or increased self-confidence. Be sure to record all observations carefully so that at the end of eight weeks you will have a valuable personal document in your possession.

On Saturday and Sunday, it can be especially challenging to keep a steady schedule. Without work, people tend to stay up late partying, studying, lazing around - or whatever fills that void. It's like some kind of law of human nature that these two days must be left empty. Don't feel the need to scramble on weekends; rather, be flexible and squeeze in 30 minutes somewhere on either Saturday or Sunday. Just remember: continuity must be maintained; so, a morning walker may choose to go for an afternoon or evening walk on these days as well. Make every effort necessary for your eight week program to be a success. A walk buddy can be invaluable during tough times; try to find one and maintain it long term for mutual benefits. Congratulations on completing your first week of walking every alternate day for at least thirty minutes per day - an achievement which may have seemed unusual at the start. Give yourself and your buddy a pat on the back; now go forth and keep walking!

Before we conclude this chapter, let us review. Fitness isn't always determined by your body type; rather, your activity level directly relates to how fit you feel. Get on track towards lifelong fitness by doing activities such as walking, running, cycling and swimming. If an irregular or non-exerciser devotes half an hour every day for eight weeks to walking, the results will be nothing less than miraculous on both psychological and physiological levels. Two wise long term strategies are to keep a walk journal and find an accountability partner for your walks. Remember to warm up and cool down properly before and after each session of walking. Snacking on light snacks/drinks prior to walking helps fuel your body but never overload it; breathe from your diaphragm and listen closely to what your body is telling you through major and minor signals.

At first sight, it might look like any old boring office with four walls but when the dust settles you'll realize there's much more going on beneath that surface!

Week 2

Now that you have completed one week of walking, it is time to focus on other important aspects of your fitness plan: arm swinging and hip-swinging as well as stretching and exercises. These last two topics will only be briefly touched upon here but are fully discussed at the end of this book. Let's begin with stretching. Here we will examine its role in daily routine. While some people opt for a pre-walk stretching regimen, it may not be recommended - particularly during colder climates when muscles need time to warm up before vigorous stretching can take place. Therefore, when walking first thing in the morning, stretch after warming up or midway through your walk and towards the end. Flexibility is essential for fitness and must be maintained over time for maximum benefit. Stretching is important, but yoga also plays a significant role in maintaining flexibility. Yoga has long been proven to not only maintain but also increase flexibility holistically. Even basic asanas can be learned and practiced easily enough; this week we won't focus solely on yoga; once our walk routine has been established, we can focus on all-round fitness goals.

Strength building exercises are essential for building muscles, whether they be used for locomotion or stabilization purposes. At the end of this book you'll find a general program for building muscular strength across your entire body; however, due to individual differences you may want to adjust it according to your own requirements as one size does not fit all.

Let's now focus on the swing of an arm. As you begin your daily walks, you may have noticed that the range of motion for your arms decreases when walking slowly. Since speed and swing are inextricably linked, you can utilize their relationship intentionally by swinging them quickly at their rise and naturally bend at your elbows. Doing this will increase both speed and distance covered within a given period of time.

The secret to walking fast lies in its technique. Slow walks are centered on your knees, while fast ones originate from your hips. As you want to increase your speed, start walking from your hips - that is, bring them into play and let them drive your steps instead of having them driven from around your knees. Intention is key. Set yourself the goal of walking fast, then act according to that intention and you will notice a dramatic improvement in both your technique and speed while walking. Your intentions should drive all decisions you make during each day's walk. With commitment and determination, you will see results! The second week is an ideal time to begin learning your new technique, as it takes two weeks to master it fully. By the end of your third week, you should be fully confident and prepared for greater levels of walking. Combining both of these concepts, walking from your hips and swinging your arms in sync with each step, results in an efficient walk. Furthermore, this ensures that you are loading your heart and lungs - two key organs for aerobic exercises - appropriately so they grow and perform more optimally over time.

Routine for Week Two

Monday Tuesday Wednesday Thursday Friday Saturday Sunday

Walk 30 minutes. Rest for 30 minutes. Repeat as necessary throughout the day until complete.

In the second week, our goal is to continue walking for the time set in the first week and also increase distance covered through increased speed. Be sure to record all details in a journal; the distance covered column from both weeks will help compare progress in technique and speed. Moreover, increase difficulty level of alternate day walk routine by placing two consecutive walks together twice; gradual overload will prepare muscles and lungs for exercise.

Week 3

After walking for two consecutive days, we now spread it out over five consecutive days with one rest day and then transition into an everyday walk routine from the fourth week onwards. Just as with Week 2, aim for greater distance covered while keeping time constant; even if it's twenty-five meters in every ten minutes! Keep a record and track your progress closely if possible; remember that walking faster and for longer distances at once puts undue strain on muscles, lungs and heart which requires gradual development over time.

Routine: Week 3

Monday Tuesday Wednesday Thursday Friday Saturday Sunday

Walk 30 minutes. Rest for 30 minutes after each walk.

As we enter week three of our walk, let's examine what you eat throughout the day. Metabolically speaking, meals at three hour intervals are ideal; so if you sleep for eight hours each night, five to six meals would be optimal for you in a day. Furthermore, there is much wisdom in the old adage: "Breakfast like a king, lunch like a prince and dine like a pauper." Start your day off right by having an abundant breakfast of carbohydrates, proteins and nutrients; remember: fresh food always tastes best rather than food that has been stored or canned for later use. As a general guideline, steer clear of junk food such as chips, deep-fried food, alcoholic beverages and ice cream with empty calories that don't provide essential nutrients. Natural food is always preferable to its processed variants; home grown organic vegetables and fruits are the highest quality options available. For a more detailed treatment of nutrition, there is a chapter dedicated to it near the end of this book.

Week 4

As we near the midpoint of this program, it is time to assess what has been accomplished thus far and plan for what comes next. You have been walking six days a week already; now complete all seven weeks by walking. Walking is an activity that can be tailored for every day of the week. From the fourth week on, walk for at least thirty minutes each day until you reach the last day of your last week - that is, fifty-sixth day). Now you are looking at twenty-eight days with thirty minutes of walking per day (plus an additional ten for warmup and cooldown). That adds up to eight hundred and forty minutes of exercise - though this may seem intimidating to those unfamiliar with walking, it won't be a challenge for you! Your first three weeks have already given you a taste of what to come if you look back and review your walk journal (if you started and maintained it religiously), you will discover that you have already logged over 444 minutes walking each week. In just the fourth week alone, however, you are on track to cover half as many miles as before! How exciting!

Now is the perfect time to introduce some novelty into your program. Consider adopting a strategy commonly used among runners: fartlek. This word literally translates as "speed play", in which either speed or terrain are varied. One round or a certain distance may be covered at faster than average speed, then the person returns to their base speed before alternating with faster variants. Or, from one kind of walking surface to another (e.g., from sidewalk to ground), walking may switch directions. Fartlek can easily be integrated into your walking regimen. It offers numerous physiological and psychological advantages, such as providing your muscles with a necessary "jolt," or overload, so they're motivated to perform better at short notice. By simulating life, walking has the added bonus of imparting its benefits onto others. After four weeks of consistent walking, a change is necessary to keep interest and optimism high in your walk. Alternating higher speed with slower average speeds helps prevent boredom by providing variety.

Routine for Week 4

Monday Tuesday Wednesday Thursday Friday Saturday Sunday

Walk 30 minutes. Walk 30 minutes more. Walk an additional 30 minutes after that. Walk 30 minutes more again before resting for 30 minutes, taking another walk of 30 minutes after resting. Walk 30 minutes more after walking 30 minutes has elapsed since your last walk and resting 15 minutes afterwards.

Though the schedule given may appear straightforward, fartlek driving makes for an exciting and varied week. As you record both time and distance covered, you will soon realize that you have covered more ground in less time than ever before!

In addition to your exercise time schedule, it is also important to be aware of other opportunities for physical activities. It helps you maintain an awareness of the daily rhythm of your life and identify spots where physical activity can be added in. Modern urban culture has made people increasingly inactive, which leads to physical inactivity becoming a natural habit. You have taken action and taken positive steps for both your physical health and mental well-being - an admirable step that I must congratulate you for. Remember not to just sit when your couch invites you to lie down and watch TV; stand when possible and walk short distances when riding or driving is easier - all these activities help your body remain active and flexible. With that in mind, let's dedicate some time for yoga!

As mentioned at the start of week two, we'll now examine the holistic yogic practice of

Sun Salute (Surya Namaskar). This series of asanas (yogic poses) must be performed in a specific order and for an extended period of time every day at least. A straightforward step-by-step method for performing it is provided below.

Step 1: Start in namaskara pose on a mat or grass, holding your hands in the pose with backbone erect.

Step 2: Raise arms overhead and lock elbows.

Step 3: Now bend at the hips without bending knees and touch your feet with hands.

Step 4: Take one foot back and keep your head straight to achieve a lunge posture.

Step 5: Now hold both arms at shoulder width before you, taking one leg back, keeping both hips up in an inverted "V" pattern at your hips.

Step 6: Bend your chest towards the ground/mat, keeping the "V" formed until both your chest and knees touch it.

Step 7: Raise your chest and head upwards while unfolding the legs so they are almost parallel to the ground. This marks midway in our 12-step process; all subsequent poses will be mirror images of each other, going backwards from step 5 back to step 1.

Step 8: Return to the inverted "V" position of step 5.

Step 9: Take one foot back and keep your head straight in order to achieve lunge posture.

Step 10: Now bend at the hips without bending knees and touch your feet with hands.

Step 11: Raise arms overhead and lock elbows for stability.

Step 12: As in the namaskara pose, stand with your hands clasped together and your back bone erect.

Once a cycle of the Sun Salute is complete, depending on one's stamina and availability, one set can consist of five to twelve such cycles. As you can see, each series of steps helps stretch muscles and joints while providing bodyweight strength training exercises at the same time. Forming "V"s or push up like movements works out chest, back and abdominal muscles; lunges provide good leg exercise as well. Through all other moves included within this cycle you are stretching one entire set of muscles twice for added benefit!

One effective way to incorporate the Sun Salute into your program is by starting with two sets per day at the end of your walk. One set means going from step one to step twelve once. Gradually, increase the number of steps one set at a time until it reaches the recommended range. The combination of walking and sun salute does several things within less than three-quarters of an hour: stretching muscles, exercising lungs and cardiovascular systems.

Week 5

Now that you have reached the fifth week of your walks, it shows that you are dedicated and determined. Furthermore, it shows us that now you are walking thirty minutes each day for seven days a week - turning physical activity into exercise! Your routine for this week will remain similar to the fourth one with added fartlek excitement added in. Additionally, feel free to alter time or distance details slightly; after all, "alter" means increase!

Routine: Week 5

Monday Tuesday Wednesday Thursday Friday Saturday and Sunday: Walk for 30 minutes; relax for 30 minutes afterwards, take a short shower, and stretch your muscles - then proceed on with your stroll!

Walk 30 minutes, rest for 15 minutes, walk another 30 minutes for another break and stretch some more before returning home for dinner and refreshments! Walk 30 minutes without stopping! Walk 30 minutes continuously...walk 30 minutes with us...walk 30 minutes...rest 15 minutes! Walk 30 minutes without stopping! Walk 30 minutes during lunch for additional exercise...rest 30 minutes! Walk 30 min before taking a leisurely leisurely leisurely leisurely!

Walking, like any other exercise, burns calories and that burns the stored body fat. This fact alone suggests that for those who struggle with weight issues, walking could be an effective means of losing pounds and improving fitness levels. But how exactly does this happen? Research shows us that taking a 30-45 minute brisk walk each day not only increases physical fitness levels, but it has been linked to greater longevity and decreased risks of many diseases as well.

Your daily regimen now includes a 30-minute walk (twenty minutes plus five for warm up and cool down). We'll cover all the other benefits in another chapter; in this one we'll focus on its effects on body weight.

By looking at the simple formula for calorie gain, it can be determined as follows:

Calorie gain = Calories consumed through food + Calories burned metabolically

Negative values indicate calorie loss or gain over an extended period. Conversely, positive numbers signify weight loss over a similar timeframe. When both variables on the right are controlled and altered, the overall impact on weight change is huge. Thus, for regular exercisers, both losing and gaining weight will only require careful calculation and dedication to reach success. If you want to lose weight through walking, all that's necessary is for you to eat sensibly and exercise regularly so that your metabolism burns more calories than what you consume. People who regularly exercise have their systems set up so they can burn calories even when doing nothing at all. Gaining weight while exercising presents a simple mathematical problem for those who wish to maximize their metabolism. They simply need to follow the formula provided above and consume more calories than they expend. Exercisers will benefit from increased muscle mass rather than fat, compared to non-exercisers. This difference in quality of weight gained would be even more evident if they had included resistance or strength training into their routine.

BMI = Weight

Here, W is your weight in kilograms and H is your height in meters. To calculate your BMI, all you have to do is multiply W (your weight in kilograms) by H2 (your height in meters squared), as shown below: For someone weighing 66 kilograms and standing 169 centimeters, their BMI would be: 66/(1.699X1.69) Kg.m-2, or 231. A simple example would have sufficed if we didn't need to understand the concept in depth; however, considering its importance throughout our program, a more detailed discussion is warranted. Research has determined that the BMI range best for health and longevity is between 20-25. A BMI below twenty or above 25 indicates either an excessively thin individual or someone who is severely overweight. Furthermore, those whose BMI exceeds the recommended range have a higher mortality rate than those whose BMI falls within it - especially for values above 40. BMI values between 25-30 are considered low risk, 30-40 moderate and above forty high risk for mortality. To illustrate this point, we have created two tables and accompanying charts; the first set keeps the height of each person constant while the second keeps their weight constant.

Chapter 3: Weight (in kg) Height (in meters) BMI

1 56 1.69 19.6

2 66 1.69 23.1

3 76 1.69 26.6

4 86 1.69 30.1.

As can be seen from the table above, a person whose height is 169 centimeters and body weight of 66 kilograms falls well within the recommended BMI range of 20-25. All other BMI values in the table yield BMI values in red indicating they are either below or above required values. Therefore, it would be recommended for someone of height 169 centimeters to keep their body weight between 57-71.1 kilograms and BMI between 24-25.

II. Calculated BMI Calculations at Constant Weight

As is evident from the table above, if someone weighs 66 kilograms and stands at height 169 centimeter, their BMI falls well within the 20-25 range. Conversely, those whose height are 162.5 to 182 centimeter will fall within a safe BMI value range.

Metabolism is genetically determined, but physical training over a sustained period of time has the power to alter it. So no matter your body type or how efficiently and quickly your metabolism burns fuel during walks, with regular exercise you can increase or decrease weight and bring it within healthy limits of BMI (body mass index). As long as you invest time into walking for exercise each day, even small changes like increased walking speed or greater distance covered will make a difference in how often and effectively the scale reads "BMI."

You have been keeping a walk journal, recording data regarding time given and distance covered each day. Furthermore, you have also recorded your weight on Monday mornings of every week. Now is the time to expand on these details in your Nutrition Journal - refer to the chapter on nutrition at the end for guidance. New columns for Calories, Fat, protein and carbohydrate intake will be introduced into the journal starting with Week 5, creating an organized table similar to what is found there for reference.

Week 6

This week's routine remains unchanged from last week:

Routine: Week 6

Monday Tuesday Wednesday Thursday Friday Saturday Sunday

Walk 30 minutes. Walk 30 minutes more. Walk 30 minutes more. Walk 30 minutes more. Walk 30 minutes more. Walking is important! Walk for 30 minutes every day this week to maintain physical fitness levels. Walk for 30 minutes on each of those days (ie: every morning!) or run for 30 seconds every other hour until complete fatigue has been overcome - that's one mile!

As you know, this is your third week of walking seven days a week. Your commitment is commendable and we need to maintain that level until the eighth week and beyond. Exercise of any kind; be it aerobic or anaerobic - has long-term consequences on human body; these impacts accumulate over time as the benefits accrue. As walks are aerobic in nature, they primarily impact lungs and heart in the long run.

It may have been challenging at times to maintain a steady pace for twenty continuous minutes, but you have been keeping yourself physically active nonetheless. By adhering to the basics outlined in the Physical Activity Pyramid and stretching daily, as well as strengthening your muscles with strength training, you are following through on its promises of improved physical activities and fitness levels. Look back at your pre-start level of physical activities and fitness and compare that with today's; chances are you have been making excellent use of your time!

Now in your sixth week of walking, only two weeks away from completing the entire program, there are no additional guidelines needed. Simply adhere to the general outline and add in some creative touches for an even better walk experience. Maintain your regular schedule, and the momentum will carry you into the eighth week. Now is the time for us to look deeper within and observe the internal changes that accompany a happy change in your level of activities. Now is the time to assess the long-term consequences of what you started six weeks ago when you committed yourself to reading this book. With confidence, I am certain that we can successfully complete this program together. So confident am I that by the end of this program in six weeks, you will have implemented the changes you find beneficial to your everyday life. I'm certain you will see those benefits reappearing in your daily life as well. Doing the aforementioned thirty minutes of physical activity a day, with planned breaks throughout the year, with planned breaks included, is what motivates you to keep on walking? Your answer may be that "that in itself is enough reward". I wholeheartedly concur!

Anyone who has ever participated in walking or running regularly knows that these activities have the power to naturally boost one's mood. Even if you started at your lowest point of energy, by the end of your session you feel energized and refreshed--especially when pushing yourself beyond what was comfortable during the journey. It has been scientifically proven that certain hormones released deep within lead to feelings of happiness - so what more do we need?

Exercise not only brings you joy, but it can also give you a better chance at living an extended and healthier life. It's like holding the philosopher's stone in your hands - exercise is not some magical elixir but rather real, life-extending power that ensures longevity. Exercise can extend and enhance the quality of your life, providing you with satisfaction and joy in return. While time does pass and we all age eventually, exercise has the capacity to delay some of the negative effects associated with aging. Exercise helps combat these wears-and-tears while increasing vitality and vitality throughout our later years. It's well known that muscle mass, strength, flexibility, speed and efficiency of our internal organic functions - even body composition - diminish with age. Although 30 minutes of vigorous walking a day may not sound like much, but it does have magical powers: It keeps you fit! How? This walk burns around 2000 calories each week, giving you an edge over non-exercisers such as your former self.

Studies conducted over time have revealed a distinct pattern in how people age. Furthermore, their internal organ structures and functioning differ considerably between individuals. Exercisers who engage in endurance training experience thicker ventricles of their heart than non-exercisers. Furthermore, regular exercisers have a different basal metabolic rate and oxygen utilization capacity than non-exercisers. The way our lungs take in and push out air is different, as are our muscles and bones. By adding resistance training into their daily regimen, people can combat the effects of normal ageing on muscle loss as well as bone brittleness or breaking in old age.

Week 7

Congratulations on completing six weeks of walking! Your routine remains unchanged for this seventh week as follows:

Routine: Week 7

Monday Tuesday Wednesday Thursday Friday Saturday Sunday

Walk 30 minutes. Walk 30 minutes. Walk 30 minutes. Walk 30 minutes. Walk 30 minutes. Walk 30 minutes. Walk 30 minutes. Walk 30 minutes. Walk 30 minutes.

At the end of your first week, I'm sure you remember feeling heavy at your shins after walking! Your mind might have told you to give up but instead, you pressed on. No one ever told you "no!" You kept walking regardless. You were determined not to quit! Despite all this, you kept walking forward. Your shin splint was gone. Your leg muscles took the strain in stride. Your lungs learned to take in as much oxygen as necessary for cell health, and exhale carbon-di-oxide efficiently. Your heart has adjusted to beat in rhythm with your body and returned to its usual level of activity soon after you finished walking. You may have also noticed that your immune system had become stronger over the weeks as a result of all this exercise. Not only do you feel good during and after each walk, but its effects last throughout the day - you have become an entirely different person altogether! All these benefits had been involuntary and unconscious; now is time for conscious effort.

Before we dive in, here are a few tips for long-term health:

Avoid smoking; quit if you do.

No junk food and no supplements.

Steer clear of drugs.

Eat clean and organic whenever possible.

Reduce your alcohol and caffeine intakes.

Abstain from hormone injections.

If you're looking to drink in excess, H2O is your answer! After six weeks of this program, all the physical and physiological elements have become integrated and naturalized in your walk. Had I discussed this earlier on in the process, you might have found it distracting or burdensome. Now, this can be quite interesting. What I want you to do is add mental and spiritual components to the physical act of walking. Take time out of each day for introspecting; even if you do so naturally and unplanned, be aware of both the process itself as well as your inner self. Besides, walking regularly not only rejuvenates physical, mental, and spiritual energy levels - it should become an everyday ritual!

Week 8

Finally, the end is here! This week will follow a similar routine as that of previous weeks. Here is your weekly itinerary:

Routine: Week 8

Monday Tuesday Wednesday Thursday Friday Saturday Sunday

Walk 30 minutes. Walk 30 minutes. Walk 30 minutes. Walk 30 minutes.

It's the last week of our program! In just six more days, it will be over. It was good that we focused on so many important issues over the previous seven weeks; some of which you can see listed on previous pages:

Maintain Your Walk and Nutrition Journals

Avoid dependence on gadgets and mechanical devices.

Be consistent and committed.

Remember the fundamentals of exercise physiology.

Monitor your meals for nutrition purposes.

Stretch properly for flexibility.

Build muscle strength through strength exercises.

Practice diaphragmatic breathing to relax.

Stay flexible by having a walking buddy along for company.

Introduce variety through speed play activities.

Follow both Pyramids - Physical Activity Pyramid and Food Pyramid!

Calculate your BMI and maintain it within the desired range.

Pay attention to your body's rhythmic movements.

Fitness isn't just having strong lungs and hearts - it also includes having a flexible body, strong bones and powerful muscles. Don't just stop there; add in yoga for strength as well - sun salute sets will demonstrate its effectiveness! Resistance training for muscles has also been proven to be the best form of fitness; studies show it must be balanced between aerobics and anaerobics for true holistic fitness benefits. For this reason, holistic fitness requires not just aerobic but anaerobic components too - the ideal regimes incorporate both types of exercises into one holistic program with proper nutrition for maximum benefits. Walking, stretching, resistance/strength training as well as proper nutrition - are all equally essential components to living a fit life!

Exercise may have provided you with a sense of euphoria after crossing half an hour mark at moderate or intense activity level. The reason behind this sensation lies in endorphin, which gives body the capacity to tolerate pain and perform under stress; plus it gives mind the capacity to resist anxiety, uncertainty and fear. Collectively it acts like an internalized opium compound - endorphins.

Endorphins that remain in the bloodstream have an immense effect on body and mind, often leading to what is known as an addiction to exercise. For those dedicated to physical fitness and holistic health, even hearing the word addiction can send chills down their spine; but in this rare circumstance - an addiction to exercising every day for a specific duration - could possibly be seen as beneficial. After all, who in their right mind would call that bad?

Chapter 4: After the Eighth Week

Congratulations! You have successfully completed the whole program. Your perseverance and intelligence in selecting the right thing have been rewarded; perseverance by sticking with it. It hasn't always been easy, but it has been an incredibly rewarding journey. Only an early morning walker understands the struggle of leaving bed when the alarm sounds early in winter morning; late afternoon walkers know the difficulty in carving time out from their busy day's schedule for exercise; evening walker have taken half an hour away from family obligations for their walk - no wonder we all find motivation through fitness together!

Change is the one constant in nature - and fitness should never be exception to that rule! To stay motivated and improve both physical and mental wellbeing, keep mixing up the routine. Walking has already given you a greater level of physical fitness after eight weeks; now it's time to add some variety into your exercise regime with some equally effective alternatives:

1. Maintain your walking routine with additional weights

II. Graduate to cross country walks, hiking or trekking

III. Try running for eight weeks

IV. Cycle for eight weeks

V. Swimming for eight weeks

VI. Engage in a physical activity that works the whole body.

Let's examine each option one by one. The most obvious choice is weights in hand or strapping them onto your body, or carrying some in a back pack, can add resistance and make walking longer more interesting by increasing the level of effort put in by carrying weights. Carrying dumbbells of one kilogram each could easily overload your musculoskeletal system and put undue strain on heart and lungs; changing up the weight carried also alters its intensity considerably, making for an exciting journey!

Cross country walking involves traversing fields or open country. A hike is a longer walk in the countryside, while trekking requires more commitment over several days. Only experienced walkers can progress from cross country to trekking; regular people cannot do both at once. Furthermore, these activities tend to work better together with friends or group; by the end of eight weeks you should have made some new acquaintances who share similar interests and goals. Now is your time to push yourself beyond your comfort zone and discover new limits!

Human bodies are amazing systems. If left unchallenged, your body becomes stronger and better at what it does. Once accustomed to walking for thirty minutes, add weights or follow more demanding forms of the same activity until it takes an additional half hour to burn the same number of calories as walking does. Running also takes less time than other exercises while still challenging your heart and lungs more - perfect if time is limited!

People with limitations or reservations about running may prefer an outdoor bicycle instead of a stationary training bicycle. Although not as taxing or effective, this alternative puts less strain on joints by distributing weight evenly over the bike. Plus, pedaling against whatever air currents are present outdoors makes for an even healthier alternative that still gets you moving!

Swimming is the ultimate cardiovascular exercise, offering benefits over running and cycling alike. In Rocky III, Apollo Creed famously said that swimming works muscles you didn't even know you had! He couldn't be more right! Swimming in its freestyle form requires pedaling with legs and cutting water with muscles of your arms, chest, back and shoulders. Even your neck muscles get worked when you turn sideways against the force of water to inhale. Furthermore, this exercise keeps your body nearly horizontal which means reduced pressure on joints. Therefore, it's an ideal exercise for overweight individuals or those with limited joint mobility. The only caveat to this great workout is that in winter or cold climates you must use an indoor pool in order to continue.

The last options on the list are sports that involve a great deal of running and utilize major muscles in the upper body - like rugby or hockey. Badminton, tennis and squash can help build stamina but place too much emphasis on arms (especially around the elbows), neglecting other parts of the upper body which leads to overuse over time - especially around elbow and wrist joints. One good game of full body sports each day should be sufficient enough to keep physical fitness at its highest level.

Be wise, choose freely - but do something! A lifelong dedication to exercise translates into an extended period of fitness and health that also improves quality of life. Before I part ways with you, one last thing should be mentioned - and what better place than at the end? My own practical advice, supported by scientific evidence. You may have noticed in yourself and others that discontinuing exercise of any kind leads to loss of body conditioning, power and performance - known as detraining. Detraining is the opposite of training; once you stop following an exercise regimen, all gains made during that period start vanishing rapidly after only one week has passed since beginning your workout regimen.

Never abandon your regimen completely. If you must ease off or need to take a break, do so without fail - just remember to keep a lighter and less challenging version of the old routine functioning at all times. Otherwise all that hard work over eight weeks with all its rewards could go to waste. If walking regularly isn't feasible, break it up into smaller chunks; thirty minutes at once may not be feasible so split up the walk time into three sessions of ten minutes each - they won't be exactly equal but 3X10min will still benefit you greatly. Likewise with resistance training: if maintaining the prescribed regime is impossible, at least try doing it once per week.

Stretching for Walk

Stretching is an integral component of exercise, and walking as an exercise offers plenty of opportunity for it. It involves intense physical activity that places significant strain on the musculoskeletal system. To keep muscles and joints flexible and ready for the next circuit, walkers and runners should perform some basic stretching exercises before, during or after their activity. Here are some simple yet effective stretches that walkers and runners can do before, during, or after exercising. Stretching for the lower body and upper body are subdivided into those for either of those: shoulders, arms, chest and back; while hips, thighs, inner thighs and calves require attention on the lower end. Before we dive in though there's one important point about stretching: never make haste nor be abrupt when doing it - this could damage muscles instead of benefiting them.

Before we dive into the details of stretching, let's first identify our major muscles that will be targeted during our walk, stretching and exercise. For convenience we'll divide up the human body into upper and lower sections with the navel as our midpoint; all muscles above it belong in the upper body while those below form part of each lower half. There are numerous excellent books and websites on muscles; feel free to consult them if you require further understanding. At present we'll keep it short and focused on our activity by beginning at the neck and working our way up through shin muscles.

Let's begin with the muscles of the upper body. Neck muscles serve to stabilize and protect the neck part of the vertebral column. Next up are shoulder muscles; there are two primary groups: trapezium and deltoids. Trapezium, Deltoids and Pectorals form the main body of the chest; serratus lies on either side for added definition. The triangular-shaped muscle protrudes above and around the shoulder joint in a distinctive fashion. Latissimus dorsii is the wing-like muscle of the back that extends from beneath the deltoids nearly to waistline. Another deep grouping in this region are called rhomboid muscles; these form the core of middle back. Finally, three major groups make up abdominal muscles. The six-pack is composed of the rectus abdominis (front/straight abdominals), lower abdominals and sides of abdomen with oblique muscles. In the upper arms there are major muscles from within and without: biceps and triceps on inside/outside arm as well as minor ones on both sides for added definition. We won't discuss minor upper body muscle groups here.

The lower body begins at the hips and moves downward; hip muscles follow followed by leg muscles. The largest leg muscle in front is called quadriceps, while on opposite side of upper leg it's called hamstring. Calf muscle is cup shaped in lower legs while many more surrounding shin bones provide support and tension on it. By knowing these names we can better relate which part of the body needs stretching with which muscle.

Stretching Upper Body With Knowledge

Neck: To warm up your muscles for walking, stretch from your neck downwards. Look to one side and hold that position for nearly thirty seconds, then switch sides.

Shoulders and Arms: Swinging your arms is an integral part of walking, so stretching both shoulders and arms together is important for good form. To do so, try this holistic stretch that's adapted from an asana in Yoga: Place the tips of your four fingers together, one palm facing and the other against your body. Lift these locked palms up so they are overhead and your entire body is stretched out like the stem of a palm tree. Stay in this position for some time. Repetit the stretch five times. There is another way to stretch your shoulders and arms: interlock your fingers behind your back near the derriere, maintain your hold, then gradually distance the palms from your body by taking them as far back as comfortable. Stretch your triceps and deltoids with this posture. Hold for up to one minute, starting from a few seconds at the beginning. Repeat four or five times.

With experience, you may even be able to do it while walking - saving some time in the process!

Back: Hanging from a horizontal bar can provide great back and shoulder stretching. Try holding onto it for counts of ten up to sixty.

Chest: Static hold is an effective way to strengthen your pectorals. Stand near a pole or door and hold it with one hand at chest height, palm facing outward. Lean forward slowly while keeping your arms tight; bend at the elbow so that the tips of your fingers touch the side of your upper chest; repeat this process with the other arm.

Stretching Lower Body

Quadriceps: Now is the perfect time to warm up our lower body muscles by stretching the largest one first - your quadriceps. Hold something solid like a wall or tree with one hand while lifting your toes with the other; let your heels touch your hamstring as you hold for half a minute before repeating on the other leg.

Calf Muscles: Start by standing a foot and half away from a wall or tree, lean forward slowly while feeling the stretch on your calves, hold for half a minute, then return to standing position. Repeat with other calf.

Strength Building Exercises

Human life is truly a miracle. From our cells to organs and systems, the functioning of our body relies on perfect harmony between several complex systems. Strength building exercises help build these miracles! How amazing that our bodies and minds can keep working seamlessly day in and day out without our conscious involvement? You who have legs to walk on and brains to contemplate its benefits are truly blessed; it's the wise who walk the path of good living with ease! Your wise decision has been demonstrated through your long-term investment of time and energy into life. Walking is an aerobic exercise, primarily cardio-pulmonary in nature - that is, it affects lungs and hearts directly; however, the body is made up of more than just organs; therefore an activity for heart and lungs involves muscles as well as bones; it creates an organic whole from top to toe.

Walking requires the muscles of legs, hips, abdomen and lower back; therefore it makes sense to strengthen and develop those areas. However, it's important to maintain a balance between lower and upper body development for optimal benefits. Resistance training that incorporates both body-weight and additional weight training has been scientifically proven to increase bone density and muscle strength.

Chapter 5: Body Weight and Weight Training Exercises

1. Chest: do #Push Ups, dips (with barbell), bench press and deadlifts / deadlifts 3. Back (Upper and Lower): Pull Ups (picture right), barbell rows, deadlifts/deadlifts/4 arms. Curls (right arm only), #Back Dips 5, Abdomen: Planks with hands hanging off table then raise to chest level B. Lower Body 1. Quadriceps: do Body Weight Squats alongside Barbell Squats 2. Hamstrings with Romanian Deadlifts 3. Calves using #Calf Raise

Note: Exercises marked with a # sign are body-weight exercises and can be done both outdoors and indoors. Push Ups, dips, pull ups, back dips, planks, hanging leg raises, squats and calf raises are examples of bodyweight exercises that don't require gym equipment or require horizontal and parallel bars for execution.

Push Ups (#Pushups): An accessible body weight exercise that requires no equipment and can be done anywhere. The goal is to keep the body horizontally streamlined and balanced while moving it vertically up and down using your arms' strength. To complete this exercise, follow these steps:

Before anything else, your feet and hands must be placed correctly on the ground.

Keep your arms at shoulder width apart while spreading your feet nearly to that same width.

Start in a parallel position to the ground, keeping your torso firm and slightly raised.

Maintain tight abdominals and an arching back bone throughout this movement.

Bring your chest slowly towards the ground, as close to it as comfortable for you, then return to the original position.

Start with five repetitions at a time; cheating is allowed but not recommended as strict form comes with time and muscle development. Pull-ups are an excellent exercise for back muscles; alter your stance by changing distance between hands or feet between sets to focus more on one muscle group or the other. Do up to fifty reps in total, divided into five sets for extra challenge.

A.1.ii. #Dips: Another straightforward exercise that requires horizontal parallel bars. Fortunately, pull up and dips bars are no longer uncommon in parks and playgrounds - meaning as a walker you may already have access to one in your circuit! To perform this exercise properly, follow these steps:

Grip the parallel bars firmly.

Give a push to the ground with your feet, thrusting your lower body upward in one swift movement until your arms are straight and elbows locked in place.

From there, gradually lower your body until your chest is parallel to your elbows.

Pause here for a second, and then return to the starting position.

Begin by doing three sets of as many reps as you can at first; later on, switch it up for three sets of ten reps.

A.1.iii. Bench Press: Bench presses are one of the most popular exercises and build muscle groups throughout chest, arms and hips. All you need for this exercise are a bench, rack and barbell with plates - unfortunately it's hard to find circuits with free access everywhere so ideally it should be done at a gym. Follow these steps for this exercise:

Lay on the bench with your back firmly supported.

Tighten up your gluteus muscles and place both feet firmly on the floor for added support.

Grip the bar at nearly shoulder width for best results.

For your warm up set of ten reps, your grip should be firm; like you are squeezing the bar while simultaneously moving it vertically.

Unrack only the bar for this warmup set and do each rep slowly while feeling its weight spread throughout your body as you lower the bar towards your lower chest.

Be mindful not to let the bar bounce back; rather, lift it after a brief pause in its lowest position.

Move the bar slowly and carefully.

It is best to learn this skill from someone, with a spotter ready for un-racking and racking the bar. At twenty kilograms in weight, start with twelve reps with just the bar then add plates of five kilograms on both sides for more challenge. Follow Arnold's scheme of sets of twelve, ten, eight, six, four and two reps in ascending weight order.

A.2.i. #Pull Ups: Not a widely popular exercise, this requires strength to pull your entire body weight with just your arms and lats. Arnold Schwarzenegger recommends doing fifty reps per day for maximum benefit to back, shoulder, arms and abdominal muscles - easier than even pushups! To accomplish this exercise safely and effectively: Follow these steps:

Hang by a horizontal bar with your arms shoulder width apart and hold onto it with one grip: palms facing outward and thumbs locking over other fingers.

Feel the stretch in your lats (latissimus dorsi).

Pull your chest towards the bar until at least your chin crosses it.

Your final goal should be to pull up from underneath you towards the bar.

At first, you may find it challenging to complete a set of even ten reps. Arnold recommends doing as many reps as possible in one set and returning for more after some time - until your fifty reps are completed. Sets of twelve to six reps until the number is achieved or pyramid sets can help if you find it difficult to follow the flat set method.

2.ii. Barbell Rows: There are multiple variations of this exercise, but we'll focus on the Pendlay Rows. In this variation, the bar is kept on the floor after every rep and then lifted from there with palms facing you and thumbs locked into place for optimal grip. To complete this exercise, complete these steps:

Set the barbell with plate at the floor so it touches your shin.

Bend from the knees while maintaining the arch of your back bone.

Pull up on the bar towards you chest-abdomen junction without using arms muscles.

Maintain your body as parallel to the floor as possible.

Hold the bar at its highest position briefly and then let gravity take its course, sending it back towards mother earth - that is, your feet.

With heavier weights, your body may tend to rise. Up to 25 percent rise from parallel position is allowed. Perform four or five sets of six to eight reps for maximum benefit.

A.2.iii. Deadlifts: Coaches often recommend this exercise as the foundation of all strength building exercises due to its use of legs, lower back, arms, upper back, shoulders and abdominal muscles. Despite its widespread acceptance in gyms around the globe, deadlifts remain relatively underutilized. One reason may be that this exercise does not target any particular muscle group or muscle, but rather builds overall and core strength. Learning the correct form for this exercise and then maintaining it every rep is not difficult; even a slight misstep could result in permanent damage to either bones or muscles or both. To ensure you maintain correct form during each rep, follow these steps:

Establish the bar with at least fifteen kilogram plates on each side, or lighter weight plates raised over one or two that remain on the floor.

Let the bar touch your shins before you bend to lift it off of the floor.

Hold the bar with hands shoulder-width apart, palms facing body.

Bend knees, dip hips, tighten abdominals and lower back muscles before taking a deep breath.

Maintain this posture throughout the lift as you keep the bar close to your body at all times.

Continue this same trajectory and form when returning the bar to the floor.

Do three sets of five reps each with ascending weights. Holding your breath and building pressure inside the abdominal cavity has the important function of stabilizing your core; it's known as Valsalva Maneuver and its mechanism is straightforward: take a deep breath. Close your glottis (the cover of your wind pipe). Push the filled air against the walls of your abdomen and diaphragm from within. With heavier loads, this maneuver becomes increasingly important to stabilize the core. Some reports of blackouts and a momentary increase in blood pressure have been noted with this maneuver, yet no overall damage appears to have been done to the body. Strength trainers around the world support it; however, those already dealing with heart issues should avoid doing it.

3. Shoulder Exercise: The Military Press, or its simpler form the overhead press, strengthens the deltoid muscles. Unfortunately it's less popular with barbells

than dumbbells (especially Arnold's variation), so we'll do a standing barbell press instead for its greater functional benefits. To complete this exercise, follow these steps:

Hold the bar with hands shoulder width apart and feet planted firmly on the floor at shoulder width.

For greater power, take a staggered stance by placing one foot slightly behind another at an angle of forty-five degrees from one another.

Un-rack the bar and place it over your deltoid muscles.

Take a deep breath, hold it in, and lift the bar straight up.

Hold it overhead with locked elbows.

Return to the initial position.

Do five sets of 10 to 5 reps on both feet together. This press is known as the military press.

4. Arms: Curls are one of the most frequently performed exercises in an average gym. This exercise works mainly the biceps muscle (biceps mltiples), located on the inner side of your upper arm. To perform this exercise safely and effectively, follow these steps:

Hold the barbell with both arms at your sides, close to your body, and hands at shoulder width apart.

Bring it up in an arc towards your upper chest, pushing it as far as possible without moving your back.

Keep your body tight during the entire movement.

Give a squeeze to your biceps at the top of the movement, then bring it back down to its starting position.

Perform three sets of ten reps each with varying weights.

4.ii. Arms: #Back Dips: This exercise targets the muscle group that balances out biceps and triceps' function. Find a place in your circuit that is elevated nearly one foot off the ground, then follow these steps for this exercise:

Keep your hands near the derrieres, almost at shoulder width with fingers facing forward.

Your legs should remain straight in front as you lower yourself with resistance on your triceps.

For greater resistance, use two chairs or benches for additional support and try doing three sets of twenty-five reps.

5. Abdominals: #Planks: As the name implies, this exercise involves balance as if one were standing atop plank upon their limbs. Keep your backbone straight and

abdominal muscles tight throughout. To complete this exercise, perform these steps:

Start in a position similar to that for a push up, with hands on the ground and feet shoulder width apart.

Slowly raise your body up onto your elbows by holding onto this position for some time.

For beginners, twenty to thirty seconds should suffice.

A.5.ii. Abdominals: #Hanging Leg Raise is an exercise designed to challenge the strength and endurance of arms, shoulders, back, hips and abdominals with each rep. You will need a horizontal bar for this exercise so hang straight from it. Follow these steps:

Hang straight from the bar when performing this exercise

Lift your legs without bending knees as high as you can.

Bending knees is the easier variant of this exercise.

Strive for three sets with at least ten reps each set at first; then gradually increase that number up to twenty-five.

B.1.i. Quadriceps: #Body Weight Squats are an excellent exercise for leg muscles. To do this exercise effectively, follow these steps:

Stand with feet at shoulder width.

Sit down so your calf muscles touch those on the inside of your upper and lower legs, touching each other.

Standing up again, keep your backbone straight and chest unbent.

Keep your hands either locked and behind your neck or swing them as you descend and ascend.

B.1.ii. Quadriceps: Barbell Squats are widely considered as one of the top exercises for strength builders. You'll need a barbell with plates and an appropriate rack, such as what you might find at your local gym, to do this exercise properly. It should be performed three times: un-rack, squat and rack the barbell before repeating each stage. Racking or un-racking a barbell requires going under it, lifting it up, then either going to or coming from the rack to where you will squat. The movement of body for both exercises, with and without weights, remains unchanged. Be extra mindful to maintain a neutral arc of your back bone and to prevent the bar from pushing down on you or your knees buckleing under it. Spotting is recommended to minimize injury potential during squats, while racking and un-racking, as well as for providing feedback about form.

B.2. Hamstrings: Romanian Deadlifts are an exercise for the hamstring muscles that is not widely known or practiced. When done properly, its effects can be felt immediately.

To do this exercise properly, follow these steps:

Hold the bar with hands shoulder width apart, palm facing your body.

Fold your hip joint in half by bringing back the derrieres.

Let the bar travel very close to your body; stop when it crosses over your knees.

Return to a standing position.

Follow this for three sets of eight reps.

B.3. Calves: #Calf Raise: The calf muscles are some of the toughest in our body. There are two types of calf raises you can do on the field: standing and donkey. For the standing calf raise, stand with feet nearly six inches apart.

Raise both of your feet up onto your toes as high as possible, then return to the original position.

Weekly Schedule of Exercise

You have two options when it comes to exercising: either combine both activities into a circuit, or do them separately. Unfortunately, gym cannot be included in that option; only then can barbell and weight exercises be done. Assuming you walk either outside on grass or near horizontal and parallel bars, here I will first discuss body weight exercises followed by those done inside a gym setting.

Body Weight Exercise Schedule

Name of Exercise Muscle/Body Part Days

Push Ups Chest + Arms Monday/Wednesday/Friday

Dip Chest, Shoulders + Arms Tuesday/Wednesday/Friday

Pull Ups Back Monday/Wednesday/Friday

Back Dips Triceps Monday/Wednesday/Friday

Hanging Leg Raise Hips + Abdominals + Lower Back Tuesday/Thursday/Saturday

Squat Legs Tuesday/Thursday/Saturday

Calf raise Tuesday/Thursday/Saturday

Planks   Abdominals
Tuesday/Thursday/Saturday

Every alternate week, dedicate one set of muscles to work on. On Tuesdays and Thursdays (for lower body), it's the lower body (legs, lower back, abs); Monday through Friday are for upper body exercises like chests, upper backs, shoulder and arms - with all other days reserved for body weight exercises like planks abdominals. If you want to reduce resistance training days down further, opt for three sets per week: chest/back sets then shoulder/arms/legs etc..

Chapter 6: Nutrition

Eating healthily, regularly and clean is paramount for fitness seekers. Our food choices influence our longevity, health and fitness levels - raw or cooked foods contain carbohydrates, proteins, fats, vitamins, minerals and fiber that all play an integral role in maintaining optimal wellbeing. Carbohydrates are burned as energy in our cells as a source of fuel. When we perform an activity or exercise, cells burn carbohydrates stored there for energy production. Proteins serve as the basic building blocks of cells and essential for growth and repair processes. Fats are essential for cell structure and function, and can also be burned when carbohydrate reserves have been depleted. Vitamins and minerals are vital nutrients required for proper body operations; fiber or roughages help facilitate bowel movements (i.e., fiber). Water is the most essential element in human nutrition and vital for proper bodily function. Without it, we experience diminished strength and energy levels. Water must also be consumed daily through food and fluid intake.

People typically plan their diet by calculating energy intake and/or according to nutrient needs. The most efficient approach is combining both methods. An adult male of medium body and moderate level of activity typically consumes 3000 Calories daily, while a female with the same details consumes 2200 Calories daily. If calories consumed exceed their expenditure, people may begin to gain weight. If the expenditure exceeds intake, weight loss will occur. One gram of carbohydrates or protein provides 4 Calories while one gram of fat provides 9 Calories. Technically speaking, one could calculate all their energy requirements from any one of these nutrients; however, to achieve holistic development and healthy living it's important to get all these essential nutrients in your diet.

Do you remember our walk journal? You have been diligently keeping it updated throughout the years. Additionally, your Nutrition Journal tracks all your daily food details meticulously as well.

Meal Time Food Item Unit Calories Fat in Gm Carbs in gm Protein in gm Pre-walk Breakfast Post Walk Lunch Evening Snacks Dinner

Once you know the details of what you eat, knowledge is power. With this insight, you can plan and improve your current diet scientifically; however, to do this we first need to establish some basics. In the USA, the food pyramid is widely accepted as a starting point; these guidelines offer flexibility regarding portion sizes and amounts; we will customize this basic plan according to individual needs later. Below is a table outlining various nutrients, their amounts and number of servings needed each day:

The Food Pyramid

Category of Food Number of Servings Amount per Serving

Cereals 6-11 1 oz bread/1/2 cup cereal

Fruits 2-4 1/2 cups, 1 apple 1/2 banana

Vegetables 3-5 1 cup raw/1/2 cup cooked

Dairy products 2-3 1 cup.

Meat/Fish/Poultry Products

2-3 1oz meat pieces/ 1 egg and 1/2 cup beans.

Fat sparingly 1 teaspoon butter or oil and 1 tablespoon nuts.

Water

Given that the food pyramid neglects to mention water, let us dedicate a brief paragraph to it at the start of our detailed analysis of nutrients. Water is essential for our cells and deserves our full focus. Eight glasses (250 ml each glass) of water per day is sufficient for an adult with average activity levels. As activity level or temperatures and humidity increase, perspiration causes further water loss through sweat, necessitating more hydration during these times. Exercises, whether aerobic or anaerobic, all require water. Don't drink it all at once; sip on water as and when thirst strikes. Sports drinks may be beneficial but for everyday walkers nothing beats plain old H2O! Start small; opt for plain old H20O as your go-to beverage.

Carbohydrates

Cereals, vegetables (roots and tubers) and fruits are excellent sources of carbohydrates - with cereals being the most popular. Bread, rice, pasta, noodles - even pizza bases! - all provide this nutrient that should make up most of your daily calorie intake. Vegetables like potato and sweet potato as well as fruits like banana are high in carbohydrates too - some people even claim weight gain from taking such meals! It is best not to overindulge though as that could potentially increase weight gain! For healthy living though it would be best if this information wasn't shared prior to walking regularly! The table below gives an idea of carbohydrates present in some common food items.

Food	Unit	Calories	Fat in Gm	Carbs in gm	Protein in gm
Rice	1cup	204	0.44	44.08	4.2
Banana	1	105	0.39	26.95	1.29
Raisins	1/4 Cup	120	0	32	1
Dates	1	23	0.03	6.23	0.2
Mango	1	135	0.56	35.19	1.06
Apple	1	72	0.23	19.06	0.36
Orange	1	62	0.16	15.39	1.23

Carbohydrates provide essential energy to human bodies and are burned as fuel in cells. For active individuals, their percentage of carbohydrates may range anywhere from seventy percent to eighty percent; typically though, it stays between forty to fifty percent. Exercise is especially vital for those looking to either gain or shed pounds, as excess calories are converted and stored in the body when taken in excess of energy consumption. To effectively burn off stored fat, one must keep their energy consumption below expenditure levels. Walkers know the importance of carbohydrates as part of their pre-walk and pre-workout nutrition. Before embarking on your walk, provide your body with some carbohydrates so it can burn them off as fuel for your journey; don't leave it running empty!

Proteins

There are two categories of sources for proteins: animal and vegetable. Milk, dairy products, fish, poultry and meat all fall under animal sources while legumes such as soy bean etc. come under vegetable sources. Non-vegetarians get their supply from fish flesh or fowl meat along with eggs while vegetarians rely on milk and dairy products which are considered vegetarian by everyone except vegans; hence vegetarian diet plans around the world depend upon these for proteins. Soy bean is particularly high in protein content for vegetarians while legumes remain staple foods around the world.

Before we continue, keep in mind that egg is considered a complete protein diet as it supplies nearly all essential amino acids for body. Furthermore, egg is one of the most cost-effective sources of this essential nutrient. People around the world choose eggs over red or white meat due to its lighter hue versus dark meat's. When selecting between them, white meat wins out hands down; moreover, combining both types of proteins for an ideal balanced diet requires at least 50% plant proteins with more than half coming from plants.

You are an avid walker. Therefore, to ensure proper protein supply for your muscles and bones, use the following formula:

Take one gram of protein for each kilogram of body weight. That means if your weight is seventy kilograms, then you need at least seventy grams of protein in your daily diet. Furthermore, if strength building exercises have been added to your routine, extra protein is required for repair and growth of muscles - this new formula for success:

For each kilogram of body weight, take two grams of protein.

No discussion of proteins would be complete without mentioning protein shakes. I will never encourage you to opt for processed food of any kind or food supplements - raw and home cooked are the only two kinds of food recommended in this book. We follow nature's path; grow as much food as possible and go organic if possible; otherwise, avoid all food that has not been cooked at home during these eight weeks of this project that you have undertaken.

Proteins: Food Sources

Food Unit Calories Fat in Gm Carbs in gm Protein in gm

Milk 1 Cup 1 146 7.93 11.03 7.86

Soy Bean 1/2 Cup 160 7 13

Lentils 1 Cup 323 13.25 36.71 16.44

Chickpea 1 Tblspn 46 0.76 7.58 2.41

Mung Sprout 1 Cup 31 0.19 6.18 3.16

Yoghurt 1 Cup 8

Fish 1 Oz 8

Chicken Breast 8 Zg 8

Powdered milk 23 Gm 9

Fat

Fat has become a dirty word in today's body-shaming and name calling culture. It elicits more fear than any other urban legend baddie does. Yet fat is essential for our systems - just as humans come with both good and bad qualities. Fat requires us to survive. Fat is essential for proper nutritional absorption; without it, food cannot give your stomach the signal that you've had enough. And without enough fat in the system, fat soluble vitamins will not work properly or remain active. Even though sugar provides more than twice the energy of an equal combination of proteins and carbohydrates combined, that does not guarantee it will be stored as fat. That misconception should not be overlooked. Fat is also broken down into its smaller components and then absorbed by cells within. Nuts like almond and cashew nuts provide excellent sources of healthy fats -

providing more for your money in terms of nutrients and calories than butter or oil do.

Fat: Food Sources

Calorie Content of Calories in Grams Fat in grams Carbs in grams Protein grams Gluten percentage in gm gluten dosage can vary between products but generally falls between 30g/1oz cashew 30g/1 oz and 856.17g for cashew, almond 1 7 0.61 0.24 0.26g and cashew 31g/1 oz = 12.43 grams 8.56 grams 517g (with skins removed).

Chapter 7: Vitamins

Vitamins, or vital amines, are nutrients required in smaller amounts than the others we've discussed so far. That's why they're called micronutrients and their precursors macronutrients; minerals will follow later. Vitamins are necessary for the healthy functioning of the human body and its protection. A full chapter could be written about vitamins - from A and B Complex, through C and D (thank goodness not F to J!), K and even P - with eleven types in total. Vitamin B Complex alone makes up half of this grouping! Vitamins play a major role in helping our bodies fight off external enemies, and they regulate various internal processes. Eggs, milk, fish liver oils, meat, orange, carrot, guava, spinach and sunlight are all excellent sources of these vitamins. As can be seen from the variety of sources listed here, it takes many different foods to supply one's vitamin needs.

Vitamin Source

A1 Fish liver oils, egg, butter, carrot, mango.

D Fish liver oils and egg with butter.

E Vegetable oils with vegetable fats added.

K Green leafy veggies such as cauliflower or soy beans for vegetarian dishes and C Indian gooseberry/guava/orange or pineapple for dessert!

B1 Dried yeast and wheat germ;

B2 Dried yeast liver eggs legumes B5 Dry yeast liver peanuts B6 Dried wheat germ egg milk B12 Liver (goat or sheep), meat (veg) fish eggs dairy product all contained here!

Minerals

Our body requires various minerals in order to function optimally. Their importance cannot be overemphasized as they form the building blocks of bones and other hard parts, hemoglobin, enzymes and hormones;

plus they're vital constituents of cell sap where they aid in transmitting impulses.

Mineral Source

Calcium Milk and milk products, sesame seeds, amaranth.

Iron Milk, egg, meat, fish or cereals.

Common salt Iodine Iodized salt Phosphorus Milk egg meat fish or cereals phosphorus-mineral blend.

Roughage

Food's journey within our bodies begins with our mouth. It then travels through stomach and intestine where it's digested and assimilated, with any excreted material excreted out the other end. One component of food we value more than its nutrition value: fiber! Fiber acts as a binding force which facilitates bowel movement by pulling out undigested waste material more comfortably and easily.

For easier comprehension and application of the knowledge presented in this chapter, a conversion table can be utilized. 1 glass = 8 ounces = 240g

1 tablespoon = 15 grams per milliliter or 3 teaspoons

1 teaspoon = 5 grams per milliliter

4 tablespoons = 1/4 cup = 60 ml.

16 tablespoons equal one cup; 24 ml equals 8 oz; two cups are equivalent to one pint and both weigh exactly the same (480g = 1 lb).

Chapter 8: Walk With Confidence

Walking is an effortless part of life that many of us take for granted. But for busy professionals who must find a quick route and always park in the first row, walking may not be feasible due to lack of time or other commitments. After all, being a professional comes with its own set of challenges!

If you are retired, work from home, or a stay-at-home parent, you may find that while some days you have time for walking, others do not. It can be challenging to know exactly how your day will unfold when it begins and sometimes hesitant to commit to anything which won't be achievable. Maybe having no gym membership and making plans only one day out at a time prevents from committing fully; or maybe making spontaneous plans brings joy and freedom!

Maybe you're feeling low-self-esteem right now. Maybe you've experienced grief, are in a difficult phase of your life, are unemployed or have put on weight more quickly than expected. Maybe you recognize that change needs to take place but are too comfortable in your current lifestyle that you fear being shot down again. You lack energy for something new; yet deep inside you want change but can't quite figure out how to make it happen.

Do you believe that walking can improve your confidence, no matter the lifestyle you lead?

Why do elementary school students get recess every day? On the surface it seems like they need time to run around and burn off some energy before sitting back down in their chairs again, but any teacher will tell you even the brightest students learn better when they get up and move around between long study sessions.

Let's apply this concept to adults: being a professional doesn't guarantee confidence -

while you may well feel secure, being one often leads to stress about work.

Establishing a daily ritual of taking a walk at an appropriate time (most professionals prefer starting their day off with a stroll in the morning, but depending on when you get off work or what time you arrive home at night may work too) can help relax you and give you more mental clarity.

By managing something simple like walking, you are in control, responsible, and taking initiative to improve yourself. That kind of confidence boosts the spirit!

No matter if you're retired, work from home, or a stay-at-home parent, the concept of unpredictable days remains the same. Your day can be filled with unpredictable elements due to other commitments that take up much of your time.

By dedicating to walking daily or every other day in a block of time that is solely dedicated to you, you will start feeling more in control of your life. That doesn't mean other activities should cease; rather, adding something for you that you alone can control will breed confidence.

If you are going through a tough patch in life and feel the need to make changes but are unsure what they should be, take a walk around the block. Not only will it be good for your wellbeing, but taking walks helps circulate air which in turn helps move things along - potentially lifting you out of this place you find yourself in!

Confidence comes from having control, and walking can be an empowering activity that promotes health. Whether it's a quick circuit around the block or a three mile hiking trail--what matters is that you are in control of how, where, and for how long you choose to spend walking.

Application:

What area of your schedule do you have control over? You don't have to commit yet - just jot some ideas down in a journal. Write about how it would feel if this small change could bring health benefits, make you feel better, and potentially help you lose weight.

Chapter 9: Health Benefits of Walking

Walking offers numerous health benefits. On the surface, it may appear that only control, confidence and peace of mind are gained; however, these factors are more significant than we often realize. When you have control over one activity that is solely yours to do, it can improve all other daily responsibilities by giving yourself some space to focus.

After a spouse passes away, it is often recommended that widows or widowers get a dog. While this can seem like an overwhelming responsibility when you need to focus on yourself, physicians have found that those who follow this instruction tend to experience less depression because not only is the loved one taken care of by something unconditionally, but now the widow or widower also has the responsibility of taking that pup on daily or twice-daily walks.

Walking the dog allows the grieving spouse to get out of the house, into nature, meet neighbors and have companionship while also having some control over one aspect of life.

Your mindset is key when it comes to your health. Once you start acknowledging confidence, responsibility, and peace of mind over something small but manageable like walking, physicians have noticed lower blood pressure among walkers. Some speculate this is because stress has been reduced through an outlet; for others it may just be an exercise benefit; whatever the case may be, walking provides peace of mind to all who participate in it.

Other health advantages of walking include muscle toning. By walking at a slower rate than running or jogging, you have the flexibility to target different muscle groups more. Some walkers will stand on their toes for a brief stretch to loosen hamstrings; bend their knees more to strengthen calves;

take extra large steps occasionally as if lunging; or start out slowly, increase speed up until reaching home before slowing back down again.

Muscle toning or not, walking regularly has been proven to be a successful tool in weight loss. Studies have even discovered that those who walk regularly experience greater weight loss success than those who jog. Walking is generally less taxing on your body (particularly joints, skeletal system and back), making it ideal for those with limited mobility who can walk longer distances more frequently than joggers who might need to take time off due to joint pain. Walkers tend to have greater endurance than some joggers and remain active and healthy well into old age or when faced with extenuating circumstances. Walking is easy, making it a popular option for many to commit to daily or every other day walking.

Walking is the safest form of exercise, making it suitable for everyone regardless of body type or age. While weight loss doesn't happen overnight, if you walk 15-20 minutes 3-5 times a week for 20 weeks, then your metabolism will start to burn off up to 20 lbs in fat. While this may not seem like much at first glance, continuing this regimen for two years can yield incredible results!

Weight loss varies depending on how often people walk for 15-20 minutes. But the more weight you lose, the greater calorie burn during a 15-20 minute walk. This is especially beneficial for those who may think they're too overweight to begin an exercise program: as weight goes down, so does confidence levels and overall wellbeing.

Application:

Next time you go for a walk, bring along a watch or other time piece (if you have access to a smart phone, set the timer/stopwatch feature). Explore your neighborhood blocks and determine which route will take 15-20 minutes comfortably. You may find that walking in your own neighborhood is more convenient than going to the gym, but if it's easier for you to do so, get into the habit of spending 15-20 minutes on the treadmill before or after working out at the gym).

Chapter 10: What Makes for Good Walking?

Every day we walk from our house, around town, and to our cars without realizing it. Some people slouch. Others get into a habit of carrying too much weight (a large purse, arm full of books or binders, tilting to one side when carrying groceries, etc.) without realizing this has changed their walking patterns without them knowing.

Though it may not seem like it, bad habits can have an adverse effect on your walking regimen and potentially contribute to other underlying issues. To ensure you're doing this simple task correctly, let's review some guidelines for proper walking technique.

Maintain your shoulders. Kyphosis (the rounding of the upper back where your neck meets your shoulder area) is becoming more prevalent among older generations, giving off the impression of someone having a hunchback, slouching posture, leaning forward or having their body in an unhealthy downward sag. To combat this issue it's important to keep your shoulders back.

Most often this occurs due to osteoporosis, congenital disease or cancer; however you can help protect yourself in the future by not slouching while walking and keeping your shoulders back. This activity helps strengthen both shoulders and chest while keeping them from becoming concave.

Maintain your chin parallel to the ground while walking. While "holding your head high" may be seen as a sign of confidence (which we've already discussed as an element of walking), keeping your chin parallel to the ground can provide additional benefits beyond mere assurance.

Keep your head high to prevent shoulders from sagging or Kyphosis, as well as strengthen neck muscles for improved posture. Furthermore, while walking, other factors may come into play that you need to be aware of; if working out in a gym on a treadmill, keeping your head up helps keep you balanced and prevents falling off the machine.

If you're out walking in your neighborhood, keeping your head high helps keep you aware of external factors beyond your control such as cars on the road, other people walking, loose dogs or wild animals. It also keeps your focus on the goal ahead which helps maintain a steady pace.

Hold in Your Stomach. There's an old joke that when someone's picture is about to be taken, someone might say, "Suck it in" or "Hold in your stomach." By acting like someone is taking your picture or holding in your stomach to impress someone, not only will your overall health and wellness improve but also more muscles are activated during physical activity; not only will this burn calories from extra strenuous activity but tone down that midsection area which may give the illusion of losing more weight there than actually is because those areas become toned and controlled through regular practice

Select Good Footwear. It may seem obvious that having comfortable footwear when walking is essential, yet it still bears repeating. Have you ever noticed how your gait changes when wearing different shoes? For example, those wearing flip flops walk differently than those in flat sneakers like Converse All Stars; heels also differ from hiking boots and hiking shoes.

Running shoes are the ideal footwear for walking. Even though you won't be running, running shoes provide enough ankle and arch support to maintain an upright posture. Shoes with too flat of an insole don't offer enough arch support and can put undue strain on both back and leg muscles.

No one in your neighborhood should be wearing heels, as these place undue strain on the joints in their feet - particularly the toes. Even hiking boots aren't recommended (unless you're breaking them in for an outdoor adventure or backpacking trip). Running shoes provide more flexibility and breathing room to the walker's feet than other footwear does, providing them with better support and breathability.

Application:

As you take a walk, start by keeping your shoulders back and your chin parallel to the ground. Squeeze in your stomach as you go along, allowing your arms to swing with control but still in control. These changes won't happen instantly for you; but try focusing on making these modifications before they become habits.

Chapter 11: Fuel Up Before And After Your Walk?

If you're going to be carrying food around in your stomach while walking, it may not be the most comfortable for you to eat a substantial breakfast before starting your journey. On the other hand, eating nothing beforehand could also prove counterproductive as calories will be burned for weight loss purposes and you don't want to reach halfway through your walk and feel faint from hunger.

Additionally, it's essential to hydrate before and after your walk, particularly if you live near a desert or dry area, are in high humidity areas, or are walking during summer or warmer months when the sun is out. Eating properly before and after your walk helps address several dietary concerns that could otherwise go unchecked.

Before beginning to walk, it's essential to have a nutritious snack. Since most experts recommend waiting three or four hours after eating before working out, having an enormous breakfast before beginning your walk won't do much good. If you tend to skip breakfast altogether, at least drink a large glass of water and consume either some juice or fruit before heading out the door.

Other great morning snacks include cereal, low-fat yogurt, a bagel or English muffin with fruit like an apple, banana or other seasonal favorites like peaches or cantaloupe. When it comes to foods for walking before starting your walk, opt for those that contain fluids since these help hydrate you.

If you are the type of walker who prefers to take a walk after work or after dinner, vegetables and pasta/rice are great options. Avoid fried foods, burgers and soft drinks though as these don't contain enough low-fat, low-fiber components for optimal walking.

After your walk is over, enjoy some healthy treats like vegetables and pasta/rice.

When muscle toning with walking, it's essential that you consume some form of protein after your walk--generally within the first half hour. Possible options include hard boiled eggs, meats, beans, chocolate milk or protein shakes--though don't go overboard: your body only requires 10-20 grams of protein per session.

Long distance walking

Long-distance walking is not a typical occurrence, but you might decide to try it after you've been walking for some time. To prepare, start eating high carb foods about 90 minutes prior to beginning the walk and ensure that during your excursion you have plenty of water; aim for two cups per two hours of activity.

Make sure not to walk after meals

Recent studies have demonstrated that walking 15 minutes after each meal for 15 minutes, or 45 minutes at the end of the day (still 15 minutes after that last meal) can help prevent diabetes. These studies suggest that walking after eating slows or stops digestion and helps direct those calories toward activity instead of processing food with normal (or sometimes elevated) levels of insulin. It may also reduce acid/esophageal reflux symptoms since gravity works to work down stomach acid instead of sitting and letting it burn high up where it usually sits. Studies suggest walking 15 minutes after a meal may reduce acid reflux symptoms in half by this method.

Hydration is key before, during, and after your walk. Even if it's only 15 minutes around the neighborhood, don't need to bring a water bottle with you; however it is recommended that you drink at least one large glass of water before leaving and another once you arrive home. Nutritionists suggest that any time you feel thirsty you may already be dehydrated so make sure to continue drinking water until full. Furthermore, drinking more water helps reduce calorie intake which in turn helps you lose weight by cutting back on snacking cravings.

Chapter 12: Starting To Exercise?

Okay, we've discussed the health advantages of walking and how it can enhance your mindset and positively influence other areas in life. We also covered how to walk properly. Now it's time for action: intellectualizing the advantages of walking and making a mental commitment are great; but how do you actually incorporate it into your schedule without stress or difficulty? Here are a few tips:

Schedule regular breaks from work

Remember in the first chapter how you made some notes about a time in your schedule that would work for you? What days and times have those been? Do you plan to commit every day or every other day? It's okay if you don't know yet.

Physicians advise that when beginning a walking regimen, you should begin by dedicating to three times per week and gradually increase it from there. You should always plan at least one day off during this time; some personal trainers recommend not having consecutive days off since this makes it harder to resume your regular schedule after taking a break (and thus more likely for you to skip altogether).

When planning your schedule, try this:

Monday on

Tuesday off

Wednesday on

Thursday off

Friday on

Allow yourself the weekend off to do other leisure-type activities without feeling the strain of work. Even if it means more days on and one off, make sure you take Sundays off (if it fits into your schedule). Our culture encourages us to have one day off each week devoted solely to relaxation - making Sundays ideal for this purpose!

No matter when in the day it falls, take time out of work for some leisure time!

You may have already written in your journal about the best time of the day to walk, and now is the perfect time to consider when that is. Many professionals and other busy individuals choose the earliest possible moment as their walk time; it serves as a form of meditation before the day gets hectic or out of control.

Some see walking as a form of grounding and foundational time to connect to who they are. Others prefer it in the afternoon after getting home from work or evening after dinner; these individuals typically view this time of day as one of down-time, relaxation and de-stressing.

Other people might have different needs. For instance, a widow who recently adopted a puppy may need to walk three times daily

- including during the middle of the day - in order for the pup to get enough exercise. If you are someone with pets, children, or other requirements related to walking, make sure you budget your time appropriately so everyone gets what they need from it.

Just do it - no excuses!

Perhaps the best way to start walking is simply to start doing so. You can always adjust your schedule if what you've planned doesn't work out, and you always have the option of skipping a day if necessary due to special circumstances like traveling for business, vacationing with family members or any other scheduling conflicts.

You can always start walking and then realize you have poor posture; take an extra day off if health issues prevent you from walking on one day for whatever reason; but the important part is to start. There will always be an excuse why not to walk today or that you just don't feel like it. But the important thing is to get moving.

No one else can make walking work in your schedule for you; only you know what works with your lifestyle and schedule. Don't get stuck on excuses: while a walking schedule may be flexible, it still needs to be done in order to reap all its health benefits.

Tip of the Day

When you don't feel like walking when you wake up in the morning, try still going anyway. Exercise releases endorphins which make you feel better; so even if it wasn't your intention to go for a walk, eventually the body will tell you it was beneficial and grateful that it did. Of course, if illness is involved, that's something else entirely; otherwise if health is good and all around then trust that taking that first step towards bettering yourself will actually improve how good it feels afterwards too!

Chapter 13: Walking as Exercise

Now that you understand the benefits of walking, it is essential to realize how important it is to get in enough steps each day for exercise. While most recommend taking 10,000 steps per day as exercise, the correct form of walk matters more - not only will these strain your muscles but they could also wreak havoc on your health by exhausting them prematurely. Incorrect steps could cause muscle fatigue and strain which will negate all efforts at exercising altogether.

Here are a few tips which can transform walking from an exercise into an enjoyable habit:

Prepare Yourself Before Beginning any Exertion

Finding the Ideal Walking Destination

For optimal walking enjoyment, select an area with flat terrain, clear paths with no deviations, smooth surface and minimal vehicular traffic. While your neighborhood blocks may provide some options, sometimes road conditions aren't what you're after or comfortable with; then consider exploring walking options in parks or other public places within your town.

Proper footwear is essential when walking, as your feet will be under a lot of strain which could cause pain. Choose something that can handle the pressure as well as something suitable for the weather - comfort and quality should always come first.

Only drive to a park if it is absolutely necessary. Most parks are flat and serene, making walking there an effective stress reliever. If there's no city park nearby, try biking boulevards or paths on either sides of the road that have minimal ups and downs with well-maintained surfaces - these could serve as great alternatives to walking due to minimal traffic.

Shopping malls make great walking spots due to their leveled, sprawling paths and variety of paths. Plus, there are usually a few stores within reach which keep you entertained if there is something on your mind. Though large in number, the crowd is dispersed and moving. Shorelines can offer peace and serenity if you live near the ocean or other large water bodies for early morning walks.

Employees with limited time can always rely on treadmills as an alternative method of exercising.

Picking Out Your Music

Listening to music while taking a walk can be extremely comforting if you get tired of staring at trees and other sights. It is recommended to listen to inspirational and pop music to focus on other parts of life and maintain an upbeat tempo. Think about what you had for dinner last night; think about your favorite movie's plotline; but do not get distracted by something as mundane as work or complicated as life's purpose. Upbeat music keeps you walking without stress; after all, this is your chance to unwind and let loose!

Don't Shoot for the Stars

If your body has been resting for some time, starting slowly and aiming for short laps is recommended. Track your progress by making short term goals and writing them down on paper. Walking is one of the basic exercises, so there's no need to exert too much energy; a fresh body with correct posture and equipment should be able to walk for several hours without much fatigue compared to running or weightlifting exercises.

Be mentally strong

Mental strength is one of the most important and yet easiest aspects to attain when investing. Create a positive mental attitude beforehand as taking small, steady steps toward your investment can pay off in the end. Get your mind set for success before diving in headfirst - taking it slow and steady is key!

Be Patient

Walking as an exercise should be seen as a long-term change that promotes better and healthier living. Doing it for one-off fitness or weight loss goals won't provide lasting benefits and may prove ineffective.

Drink Plenty of Water

Consume at least 8-16 ounces of water an hour prior to starting your walk. Drink more if you plan on walking for longer duration or distance as this acts as a reserve and could prevent dehydration mid-trek in hot sun - an unpleasant situation! Carrying a metal water bottle makes carrying it convenient and helps keep you hydrated throughout your trek as you walk.

We advise against drinking too much water, as this may cause stomach cramps. Furthermore, know that chances of finding a bathroom while on an extended walk are slim.

Prior to embarking on your long walk, make sure your body can easily process all water consumed.

Walk In Circles

Design a path so that no matter how far away from your starting point, you can always return to it. Walking circles or an oval path for half a mile around is ideal as this minimizes the likelihood of getting lost or missing your track while walking. If it's convenient, extend your walk beyond what was set for--raise the bar! Walking is lighter on your body than other exercises so don't be afraid to push yourself further!

Time Management

Time management is essential for the smooth running of almost any activity. For walking, set a specific duration and commit to it - don't worry about how long it takes; focus on the outcome instead and just keep moving until you reach it. Starting with just 2-5 minutes each day can be an effective start, and gradually increase it over time as more convenient.

Avoid measuring how far you have walked when trying to improve your walk. Faster and farther walks will come naturally with practice.

Aim to improve the quality of each step you take while making this a habit.

Dedicate More Time

Every day or week, increase your walking time by 30 seconds to 1 minute as long as it is convenient and sustainable. It doesn't need to be consistent - just a minimum increase is enough. Set an achievable goal and track progress over time; once 10 minutes have been added on, the rate won't increase exponentially anymore; instead, gradually and steadily increase your walking distance over time.

Add More Speed

If your body can sustain 45 minutes of walking daily, increase the intensity and venture off oval tracks into city streets with faster legs. You will encounter inconsistent roads which will make walking more difficult and enable you to regulate your pace accordingly.

Continue to search out more challenging trails, and you could possibly face the ultimate challenge of hiking up hills and cliffs.

Reach your Target Heart Rate

For better accuracy and precision when walking, wear a heart rate monitor. Alternatively, measure it manually; this is when your heart starts pumping faster and you start panting. If your speed falls below your target heart rate (THR), increase it for increased effectiveness of the exercise.

Your body will start burning stored fat only if you consistently cross your THR for an extended period of time. Even mild exercises like walking won't provide noticeable results without consistent effort and sweat, not just one day or week.

Experiment

After your body gets used to a general physical routine, try experimenting with intervals. Walk at increased speeds for one to two minutes and then slow down to your normal rate for two minutes. Practice interval training every day or alternate days until you reach your desired total time including rest periods. As you become physically fitter, minimize resting times until they're down to one minute or less so that you can maintain momentum when resting instead of coming to a sudden halt.

Chapter 14: Walking Workouts

In the previous chapter, we explored how walking can be utilized as an exercise. Now let's take a closer look at different walking workouts that can help us achieve a toned physique. No matter if you want to shed pounds, boost energy levels, motivate yourself or just tone some areas of your body, body workouts are necessary for successful results.

Make the most out of every opportunity: start burning fat now!

By adding vigorous and intense walking to your daily routine, you could potentially shed pounds and inches within a month by increasing the amount of fat burned during and after cardio workouts. There are other convenient options like 10-minute morning routines for busy weekdays or indoor options for rainy weather or working professionals. For best results, commit to at least 20 minutes high-intensity walking (coupled with workouts for additional fat burning) on three alternate days per week; other days do mild or moderate activities for around 30 minutes each.

Walking Workout 1: Treadmills

Time: 30 minutes

Treadmills are ideal for working professionals who need to tone up but lack time to walk around town. There's no need to worry about weather, traffic or darkness with treadmills; plus, tracking your speed increase as you become fit is a huge motivator!

Walking Workout 2: Sprint

Time: 25 to 30 minutes

Sprinting increases distance covered and burns more fat, so the faster you walk the greater your fat burning potential. Sprinting has been known to burn as many as 175 calories in one session! Start off slowly by warming up for five minutes then go as fast as you can for about 10 minutes; remember how far you have covered! Turn around and walk back at a brisk pace but slowing down gradually so your body has time to rest; next time aim higher and farther!

Walking Workout 3: Marathon

Time: 60+ Minutes

An hour-plus walk can reduce more than five times more fat compared to a 30-minute stroll. An hour of walking could burn around 350 calories, helping you stay in shape for events such as half marathons by providing you with longer strain. Plus, it can be integrated into social events where friends meet up to walk along your route together.

Walking Workout 4: For Extra Belly Fat

This walking workout targets belly fat specifically.

Time Needed: 10+ Minutes

A high-intensity workout like this one is great for belly fat burning and can help shape those abs if you're trying to show them off! Use these tips when planning your walk:

Draw your stomach in towards your spine, trying to maintain a contraction without holding your breath. Doing this will help the muscles gain shape.

Allow your legs to move freely as one leg swings forward and back, causing the hip to pivot with it. This slight swivel causes your lower body to rotate, stretching more stomach muscles for tightening at your belly.

Walking Workout 5: Blend Everything

Time Commitment: 10 Minutes

Intense activities can be condensed into a 10-minute workout that burns 70% of body fat. This workout saves time and is perfect for people on-the-go.

Recharge Your Body and Mind

This routine can be used when you need an energy boost and lift of mood. All it takes is 10 minutes of walking for improved circulation which activates your mind; increasing it to 30 minutes could provide an 85% boost. These work as wake-up calls which last 12 hours, recharging both body and mind for further activities of the day and reaching any goal - be it losing weight, toning up or getting healthy - this workout can help.

Walking Workout 6: Stress buster

Walking Workout 6: Mood Lift

Time Commitment: 10+ Minutes

Invigorate both mind and body with this workout, commonly referred to as a 'Happiness Walk'. The longer and further you walk, the greater the benefits you'll experience.

Step 1: Focus on your feet, feel the blood flow to them and feel the firm ground beneath you. Tap it lightly a few times while maintaining awareness of your steps for two to three minutes.

Step 2: Focus on breathing in and out. Keep an upright posture, expand your chest, and inhale all of the energy that's being taken in. Exhale any toxins associated with fatigue or pain by inhaling the positive air into your lungs and cells.

Step 3: Talk to yourself. Becoming your own worst critic and motivator by thinking about breathing will help to relax you and increase attention span.

Walking Workout 7: Brainpower Booster

Time Needed: Under 20 Minutes

This kind of workout helps the body assess its hand-eye coordination. It activates the brain and some underused muscles like your outer and inner thighs. For best results, do this routine on an average school track that measures quarter mile in distance.

The Workout:

Lap 1: Begin at the beginning of the curved end of the track and walk at your warmup pace for one full lap.

Lap 2: Make a right turn onto the next track, with your right leg ahead. Shuffle around to the other part of the track and walk back on an even straight track. Finally, turn left into the bend with your left leg ahead and continue walking forward on this same straight track.

Lap 3: Here you must repeat the process used in lap 2, which was walking sideways and backward, then turning around and heading sideways towards the front.

Lap 4: Begin walking ahead and gradually slow down for a full lap, covering one mile on either a 1/4 mile path or another mile-long walk. You can practice more sets, going on for half or full sets of each type of walking.

Walking Workout 8: Hold the exercise under trees!

Time Required: 5+ minutes

Nature can bring out the best in you within minutes. Exercising outdoors (such as taking a lunchtime park walk or an all-day mountain hike) not only improves your memory and attention span, but it's much less distracting than urban city walking due to fewer distractions and is generally more relaxing).

Maintaining Your Body

Incorporating body toning exercises or techniques into your general daily routine can transform morning walks into full-on muscle building sessions. Aim for a specific tissue every week; these workouts can be done once or twice per week with related lower and upper-body routines on alternate days; avoid working on the same tissue consecutively. For maximum effectiveness, incorporate walking routines from other sections on in-between days to burn excess fat and get your muscles in shape.

Walking Workout 9: Use walking poles

Time: 25 minutes

Utilizing walking poles has been known to increase calorie burn by up to 46%, as the workout involves the whole body with correct angles of hand and shoulder for firming throughout. Plus, with their reduced shock impact on joints, using walking poles reduces shock impact on joints.

Walking Workout 10: Treadmill Butt

Time: 25 minutes

This workout keeps the speed constant throughout with gradual increases in incline. You can complete the full 25-minute routine or opt for shorter 5-minute hill climbs for a quicker session.

Walking Workout 11: Arm Shaper

Time: 20 Minutes

Warm up your body for 4 minutes with easy walking. Increase the intensity to moderate and do 25 reps of each exercise for 25 reps. When finished, tie a resistance band around your neck and speed up for a quick walk similar to when we are in a rush. Repeat these 25 reps for 20 minutes until all exercises have been completed. Calm down by taking 4 minutes easy walking; set bar higher with more difficulty by placing hands closer together so there's less resistance from the band or separate hands for greater slackness in stride.

Walking Workout 12: Butt Firmer

Time Commitment: 16+ minutes

Walking uphill burns about 25% extra muscle fibers due to faster signaling and firming than walking on flat ground, since your body is under strain as it strives forward. For best results, find a hill that takes 2 to 2 1/2 minutes to climb and give this workout a try!

The workout: This workout is an outdoor adventure. Walk at a slow pace for 5 or 10 minutes as warm-up, then climb up and down with 2 minutes of quick, brisk pacing on a flat surface. Repeat these steps to achieve firmer and better-shaped butts. Finally, finish with 5 minutes strolling to cool down.

Working Workout 13: Sculpt All Over

Time Required: 25-40 minutes

This workout will build your strength for walking and cardio exercises while toning up.

The Workout: Write out your strength moves on a piece of paper. Utilize different exercises to strengthen all important muscles, such as bench push-ups, tricep dips, lunges, walking planks and power jumps. Put these in a jar and draw them before beginning your walk. Warm up at a slow pace for 3-5 minutes then walk quickly for 5-10 minutes. Stop and do one strength move for 10 reps then continue walking quickly for another cycle until complete. Finally, relax your body by taking 5-10 minutes after finishing this workout.

Walking Workout 14: Leg Toner

Time Required: 5 Minutes

This workout is ideal for busy homebodies as it has an easy home routine and can be completed indoors. With only 5 minutes required per workout, you can do this anywhere (need stairs included!) to tone your legs in no time!

The Workout:

1. Begin by walking up and down one stair as usual, crossing your bottom foot over top and continuing your ascent with your head

up. You can repeat this step by changing the orientation of your feet.

3. Begin at the top of the first stair level and descend using your right foot in an upward motion of right up, left up, right down and then left down for about 10 times. Repeat with other foot.

4. Skip a step while going up the stairs and then quickly come down by using each one.

5. Run up the stairs and quickly walk down them quickly.

6. Repeat steps 4 and 5 four or five more times.

7. At the bottom of the stairs, keep your right foot on either the first or second step, bend your knees, and lower into a lunge. Your right knee should direct one nail in order to give an accurate signal. Do this for one cycle by starting with your right hand then switching over to your left leg and repeating this motion.

8. Enjoy a brisk walk up and down the stairs by stepping on each step precisely.

Chapter 15: Maintenance

In previous chapters, we explored how walking affects our body and how it can be utilized for exercise and working out. With increasing time on our hands, however, staying committed to a nutritious diet and regular exercise may prove challenging no matter how physically fit you are.

Especially during the holiday season, when there are often gatherings with family and plenty of delicious treats on the table, it can be especially challenging to resist your impulses. In this chapter, we'll look at ways to stay on track with your diet and maintain exercise throughout the year - especially during festive occasions.

It is a well-known fact that the average American gains two pounds during the holiday season, yet many fail to burn off this excess fat throughout the year. Over time, this excess layer of fat accumulates in tissues, giving your physique an unflattering look, as it sits dormant underneath all that festive clothing.

No amount of willpower will ever completely defeat temptation, particularly during the holidays. But you can take steps to minimize unhealthy and junk food intake that could add extra pounds. To do this, focus on strengthening your mind and becoming mentally strong with these simple strategies:

Plan ahead and prioritize tasks; always have a backup plan just in case!

Before attending a family dinner or event, make sure to eat a high-protein snack before leaving. Not only will this fill your stomach but it may also make you feel less hungry compared to a high carbohydrate snack. Consider healthier alternatives for snacks to keep yourself from starving while on the go or in class. Likewise, when hosting an event, search for healthier versions of holiday foods so both you and your guests benefit.

Avoid high calorie drinks too!

Liquid calories are just as important to a diet as what you eat. Avoid carbonated soft drinks or sweetened sodas with high carbohydrate contents; instead, drink water or red wine with club soda and lime for the same taste but a healthier choice.

Focus on something other than food while you consume calories

The holidays are a time to spend quality time with those you care about, commemorating times spent together as memories. Make memories by doing activities other than eating together - join a group, try something new at the board game table, take a walk in the park or even take yoga classes together - that focus on enjoying each other more than what food has been consumed.

Avoid binge eating during these celebrations to maximize enjoyment from what's left over.

In today's fast-paced world, stress is an unfortunately part of everyone's lives. It follows us everywhere--even to bed! When faced with stress, many turn to food for comfort - particularly during holidays when there's typically plenty available. To combat it, set aside at least 30 minutes each day--no matter how busy you may be-- for yourself; do self-motivating activities such as going for walks, meditation or reading a book-- anything that brings joy! Additionally, making time for exercise should always remain top priority during stressful situations

Avoid oversleeping and skipping your morning workout because of fatigue from the night before. This could disrupt both your schedule and sleep quality. Instead, use exercise as motivation to wake up early and fit in some physical activity into everyday situations like taking the stairs, doing sit-ups during TV commercial breaks, walking a bit farther before calling a cab, cycling to get groceries - anything! Increase your heart rate from time to time to stay fit and healthy without doing much extra effort - plus, it allows for some days off from exercising altogether!

Sleep well is key!

Staying up late and not getting enough sleep are often associated with attending social events. Unfortunately, this lack of shut-eye can have serious consequences on you in the form of weight gain, reduced immunity levels, and an increased likelihood for illness. To combat these effects, set a strict bedtime and stick to it for one month. Select important events that could keep you up later than normal but still ensure that you get adequate rest each night.

Maintain Exercise Intensity

Though not immediately noticeable, unhealthy habits have long-term repercussions that cannot be ignored. We all wish for them to change but often find the motivation or willpower necessary for making those changes; while for others, the challenge lies in trying to form new healthy routines such as exercising or eating healthier meals; these can be particularly challenging to form over time.

Establish healthy habits by understanding the motivations and obstacles in your way. Maintaining a balanced mindset is essential for creating and maintaining good habits. You must:

1. Consider why you want to exercise. A healthy and fit body can render most disease-causing organisms ineffective.

2. Recognize what obstacles stand between you and achieving a healthier you; identify these things that hold you back.

By understanding this, you're nearly there - on the path to maintaining healthy habits and getting fit. Some common motivating factors for exercising include weight loss, general health benefits, fitness level and a presentable body structure. Unfortunately, common barriers include time commitments, stress, work commitments or laziness. Here are some tips to make exercising part of your everyday life.

There are plenty of strategies and tactics you can use to help you maintain exercise as a habit:

Social support systems offer invaluable assistance in this regard.

Find someone close to you, such as a friend, family member, coach or mentor who can guide you in your efforts to break away from bad habits. If they could partner with you for exercise, both of you could motivate each other when one doesn't feel like exercising and reap the benefits together.

Make observations along the way

Record your exercise time or distance walked at various speeds. By doing this, you can set short and long term objectives which will motivate you, especially after three to four weeks when you see how far along you've come and how much more progress is possible.

Make no excuses; stay motivated!

Avoid making excuses during the first month, as your body is still adapting to the strain and any irregularities could have serious repercussions. When feeling fatigued, take a stroll and walk slowly for around five minutes - remember, the hardest part of this journey is not starting but maintaining it!

Experiment with different exercises or activities to stay motivated!

Add fun activities like walking, cycling, swimming, tennis, weights, yoga and gym classes into your workouts for a rewarding and stimulating experience. Do multiple such exercises throughout the week to avoid getting bored.

Reward yourself after each successful effort

Choose a short-term goal and work toward it. After accomplishing it, reward yourself appropriately and think progressively. Habits will take root when you consistently reinforce them at specific times in your lifestyle. Becoming more habitual involves replacing unhealthy behaviors with healthier routines.

Checkmarks! Habits will form when we positively reinforce them at specific moments throughout our day.

Chapter 16: Treadmill Practice

The treadmill was an astonishment of its time, designed by William Edward Staub, an English mechanical engineer. Originally intended to serve as punishment for slaves, modern technology has since enabled it to be a machine that provides powerful exercise options.

With treadmill running, you are in complete control and can choose your own difficulty level based on fitness levels and abilities. In case the weather conditions are unfavourable for outdoor exercise, treadmill running offers a lighter alternative that doesn't put too much strain on the body. Many treadmills come equipped with customization features which help recreate outdoor conditions while testing our bodies to their limits.

When running on the treadmill, there are a few key points to keep in mind - such as its length, frequency and intensity. By tracking these metrics you can figure out ways to experiment and add variety into your sessions without becoming bored with them. Set goals that push you beyond comfort zones yet are achievable even without assistance if needed. With regularity you should experience an increase in energy levels from this practice!

Difficulty Level: Anything that challenges you

Time Required: At least 30 minutes

Getting Started

1. Determine the length and intensity of your treadmill runs

2. Incorporate both extreme and casual exercises 3. Identify ways to add variety into each session while knowing when it is time to stop experimenting

4. Create a schedule with adequate rest hours in between each workout

5. Prepare your body both physically and mentally before and after each workout

6. Record observations and keep a record

Note: * You might want to consider investing in your own treadmill * Use an effective pace

* Seek additional assistance from a physiologist If needed.

Plan the duration and intensity of your treadmill runs beforehand.

Length of Workout

Your workout intensity and duration depends on how well you manage time. National Institutes of Health has recommended a 30 minute workout period five times a week as the recommended standard for young individuals. You may vary this according to your daily body practice and intensity per session.

Workout Duration

Calculate the number of calories your body requires to function optimally. This way, you can decide how many are necessary to maintain or lose weight. There is an optimal calorie intake which varies based on age, activity level and whether you wish to lose, maintain or gain weight. Knowing your Basal Metabolic Rate (BMR) also gives insight into how much exercise is beneficial for each individual's fitness level.

Intensity

Running isn't just about speed (pace), it's about running with intensity (grade). Aim for medium to high intensity and track your exercise intensity by interpreting how much strain is necessary to reach your desired goal.

Both extreme and casual workouts can be beneficial; make sure you find what works best for you!

Speed

Walking, jogging and running are all beneficial workouts but rarely integrated together in one session. Working out should be about improving yourself; start slow with walking then gradually increase the intensity with some jogs mixed in for good measure. Generalized speed guidelines have been set for certain activities; you can always vary it to suit your preference: 3.55 for Walking; 5.0 for Jogging; 6.0 For Running

9.0+ Miles per Sprint

Incline

A treadmill can simulate an ideal track for running that's much easier than outdoor exercise. Set it to 1% incline and you'll experience resistance similar to what you would experience while outdoor running.

Advantages

Elevating your heart at a slower walking pace increases your heartbeat, with less impact on knees and hips. Plus, it keeps your spine upright which increases speed by stretching Achilles tendons and calves.

An incline is like hiking; walking at 3 mph may seem slow but it's just as taxing as maintaining a sustained 15% incline without assistance. There's increased motion at the lower body which is important for development; so set a pace and incline that suits your fitness level and enjoy this challenging exercise!

Basic Treadmill Workout - Walking Hills

Before beginning a workout, it is essential to do five minutes of warmup exercises on either an even surface or one with some elevation change.

Discover your ideal setting that pushes you with varying speed and incline but is manageable enough for 30 minutes without collapsing. If this is your first time doing the workout, remember that your calves will tire out before your lungs do - so take this into consideration when choosing which workout to try first!

As you go along, experiment with the protocol by doing faster walks at low inclines and very slow walks at higher inclines.

Finally, decide when it is time to stop experimenting and move onto other exercises.

Activity Variety

The treadmill gives you the opportunity to progress from slow walking to running. Additionally, adding breaks in your workout session allows for increased intensity variations. Create a custom program for yourself or use one of the inbuilt options to find one that meets all your needs.

Interval Workouts

Interval workouts feature changes in speed and incline that help you burn more calories, adapt, and stay focused. Each interval begins with a shift up in heartbeat during intensity changes and maintains that state for around 5 minutes before ending with a static state for resting. Choose an interval that will push you to high stress levels followed by a resting period to catch your breath.

Basic Interval Workout Tips

The speeds and inclines listed are only for a standard workout. You can go faster or slower, increase or decrease the difficulty level according to your fitness level, with intervals lasting anywhere from 30 seconds up to 10 minutes depending on the speed you choose.

The shorter the interval, the higher the intensity levels that may only last a short while. Therefore, for a one-minute interval you should feel out of breath after one minute. Recovery intervals provide calmness and relaxation so you can catch your breath; these usually last anywhere from one to five minutes.

Some treadmills come with integrated interval programs, though the range of incline changes varies by model. If you want both very high and low grades in one program, however, there will only be a 6 percent change - there is no requirement for both options.

Manual adjustment of the resistance is ideal and most accurate. Set repeat intervals at anywhere from 3 to 10 times depending on your workout duration, then follow a schedule accordingly.

Frequency should then be maintained at this level throughout each interval.

Based on the length and intensity of your workout, as well as other exercises you plan to do, you can determine how often you should run on the treadmill.

Schedule It

After gathering all your data, set a timetable for yourself to work out. Doing this will help with performance as it helps create habit of regularity; plan at least 4-5 sessions and don't skip any so that it becomes an established part of your lifestyle. Remember to leave time for resting or socializing with family/friends too; these should all have equal weighting in your schedule.

Get Ready

Now is the time to get your body in optimal condition by organizing some exercises into routines! With these steps in place, prepare yourself physically ready for success by setting an achievable timetable now!

Now get ready by getting into shape

Warm Up Before Each Work Out

A warm-up is essential for the body to prevent injuries caused by strenuous activity. The purpose of a warm-up is to raise the temperature of all parts of your body, prepping you for strenuous activity.

After each workout, it's essential to cool down. The primary aim should be to gradually decrease the intensity of aerobic activity and return the body to rest.

Cooling down plays an integral role in this process by, among other things, helping your muscles repair themselves after intense exertion.

* Preventing blood pooling by returning it back to the heart rather than allowing it to pool in muscles that cause spasms

* Gradually bringing down the heart rate back down to a normal beat

* Ensuring that the brain receives sufficient supply of blood and oxygen by breathing out properly * Avoiding lactic acid accumulation in muscles * Maintaining an accurate record

Track your activity, duration, intensity and response times. You might want to consider buying your own treadmill so that you don't have to depend on going to the gym for exercise anymore. This would save time and allow for greater control over exercise routine.

Maintaining good form

Along with the vigorous exercises, it is essential for your body to maintain proper form when using a treadmill. Doing so allows your body to reap all the benefits from the exercise as well as stabilize its form.

Look Ahead

Keep your gaze fixed on the ground 10-20 feet ahead of you. Maintain a straight and upright posture with your head high, spine straight, shoulders raised (but relaxed and symmetrical); do not hunch over.

Place both hands on your waist and begin to relax. Make sure the arms are at a 90-degree angle and just touching your hip.

Stride with a short stride to minimize impact on your legs. Land with a mid-foot strike and avoid heel striking as this could send shockwaves to sensitive nerves surrounding your legs.

Avoid Holding the Handrails

Holding onto the treadmill rails will cause you to hunch over and could potentially lead to neck, shoulder and back pain. Though this type of running may feel faster at first glance, the impact on your legs from pulling yourself may be much greater than expected. Avoid this form of exercise at all costs!

Outside running without rails can be intimidating, so try to mimic such conditions by slowing down or increasing your pace. Remember: the railings are only there to give support and are only necessary for beginners; cheating your workout by touching the rail may seem easy but becomes an addictive habit once caught; slow down rather than cheat yourself!

Chapter 17: Nutrition for Runners

Do your research before trying this at-home activity!

This chapter reviews six rules designed specifically for runners' diet.

Unfortunately, most of the eating plans offered to runners lack actual food content - they may not be starving but instead consume plenty of calories from nutrient-enhanced drinks, energy bars and zero-fat products that do not provide real nourishment. In doing so they often neglect consuming produce like vegetables, fruits, lean meats and whole grains which are much healthier alternatives to packaged goods.

Food is more than just nutrients. Our bodies require multiple molecules for proper growth and development, such as color components in fruits and vegetables, fibers from seeds, nuts, and dairy foods, etc. Consuming an entire fruit or vegetable provides you with all these necessary elements necessary for growth and development.

High-energy protein bars and drinks offer runners a convenient, yet regulated, way to get the essential nutrients. Following six rules daily will give your body all of the essentials it needs in addition to running or exercising regularly.

Seed-oriented foods

Seeds may be overlooked or given less importance than other foods, yet most seeds (including whole grains, beans and tree nuts) contain essential nutrients necessary for life - as well as health-promoting compounds. Not only do these contain essential proteins and fats, but seeds also boast bioactive antioxidant species like phenolic compounds and ferulic acid.

Research has demonstrated that consuming plant seeds can improve health and optimize body weight. Eating whole grains and beans has been found to have minimal risks of type 2 diabetes and cancer, as well as low cholesterol levels. Therefore, this dish is ideal for people who must stay active 24x7.

Ingredients for Walnut and Blueberry Bran Pancakes

** 1 1/2 cups whole milk

* 1 cup instant oats

* 3/4 cup sifted all-purpose flour

* 1/2 cup chopped walnuts

* 3/4 cup blueberries * 1/4 cup Oat Flour * 1 tablespoon baking powder * 2 tablespoons honey * Salt * 2 eggs beaten

1. Begin by placing oats, flour, baking powder and salt into a bowl. Whisk until well mixed.

2. Next add milk and eggs - whisking vigorously for several minutes - before mixing honey into the batter to ensure an even consistency.

4. Finally add walnuts and blueberries before stirring thoroughly again.

5 Finally pour out onto hot greased pan while cooking till top looks bubbly then flip.

7. Finish cooking both sides until your dish is thoroughly cooked; garnish with fresh fruits and veggies for extra enjoyment!

Eating fruits and vegetables provides your body with essential vitamins, carbohydrates, and calories for daily functioning. Not only that, but their vibrant colors such as yellow, orange, red, green, purple etc. also play an important role in providing health benefits beyond mere aesthetic appeal.

Pomegranates contain anthocyanins pigment, tomatoes lycopene pigment and carrot beta-carotene which provides vibrant orange hue. Pigments like these have been known to reduce cancer, heart disease and Alzheimer's risks while improving memory function. Furthermore, antioxidants present in these fruits or vegetables help minimize inflammation caused by disease or heavy exercise as they contain anti-oxidants.

Eating a variety of vibrant foods will be beneficial, as all these pigments need to be present and working together for maximum benefits. This explains why taking beta-carotene supplements doesn't lead to the same health benefits as consuming an array of colors at once. The following dish has all these vital pigments bound together.

Grilled Vegetable with Key Lime Chimichurri

Ingredients * 3 bell peppers of all colors chopped * 2 mushrooms quartered* 2 zucchini rounds diced* 1 onion diced

Vegetable Rub * freshly ground black pepper * 1 tablespoon dried orange rind* Salt* 1/2 teaspoon sea salt* Chili powder Green Sauce * 3 bay leaves dried* 6 garlic cloves crushed * 1 Poblano pepper chopped * 1 Serrano chili chopped * Sea Salt * 1/3 cup parsley finely chopped * 3 key limes chopped * 1/4 cup oregano oregano* 1/2 basil finely minced * 1/3 olive oil Method

1. Marinate the vegetables with the rub and set aside.

2. Preheat the grill to 250 degrees Fahrenheit.

3. To a mortar, mix garlic, pepper, bay leaves, lime juice and salt together to form a smooth paste (you may use your blender too).

4. Then transfer this paste to a mixing bowl along with all herbs - mix thoroughly.

5. Add olive oil to a bowl and whisk until completely mixed.

6. Skewer the vegetables onto skewers and grill until desired doneness.

7 To serve, top off with cooked wild rice and drizzle the sauce over for extra flavor!

Drop the Peeler

Eat plant foods with their skins intact. Most fruits and vegetables have outer layers as a protective shield from UV light radiation, parasites, and other pathogens. Scientifically speaking, these same outer layers contain numerous phytochemicals which may improve your health in various ways - for instance grape skins contain high amounts of resveratrol while onion skins possess quercetin; both compounds help lower heart disease risks, colon and prostate cancer chances, as well as strengthen your body.

Ingredients for Curried Lentils and Butternut Squash

* 1 cup dry mix lentils

* Whole Butternut squash

* 1 teaspoon chili powder

* 1 tablespoon olive oil * 1 teaspoon ginger (grated) * 1 tablespoon curry powder

* Salt * Pepper * 1/4 cup shredded coconut

Method

1. Grease a baking tray and set it aside.

2. Next, take a large pot and add lentils, covering with cold water.

3. Place over medium-high heat and bring to boil; add chunks of squash as it comes to a boil.

4. Simmer until squash is soft but still firm to the touch - about 15-20 minutes.

5 Finally, remove from heat, drain thoroughly and set aside.

6. Remove the squash chunks and mash them thoroughly.

7 Set your oven to pre-heat mode at 400 degrees Fahrenheit 8. In a large mixing bowl, mix lentils and squash together thoroughly.

8. Then add olive oil with spices, season with salt, then combine thoroughly.

10. Pour onto greased baking tray 11 and bake for 20 minutes or until done; top off with coconut if desired.

Glass of Milk

Milk products, whether from cow, goat or mammal milk (as opposed to soy milk), cheese, yogurt and kefir should all be part of any runner's diet. Milk provides calcium which serves as the backbone for bone formation and strengthening; correct alignment and structure are crucial when running.

Dairy food provides runners with plenty of protein to help absorb impact during workouts. Whey protein found in dairy foods also boosts immunity levels; most milk products contain stearic acid which has been scientifically shown to lower blood cholesterol levels. Studies also demonstrate that regular dairy consumption can lower your blood pressure. Furthermore, those who incorporate dairy into their diet tend to lose more fat than those who cut calories out altogether.

Fermented dairy products like yogurt and kefir contain live bacteria which aid in digestion as well as immunity. CLA (conjugated linolenic acid), an essential fat found in dairy, has been known to prevent constipation, reduce pain from certain intestinal problems like inflammatory bowel disease, and minimize episodes of yeast infections in women. Lactose-intolerant people can benefit from regular consumption of cultured dairy products; the following recipe offers ample amounts with plenty of these beneficial components:

Seasonal Fruit Smoothie

Ingredients: * 1/2 cup seasonal fruits * 3/4 cup low-fat yogurt* 1 cup milk* Almonds* * Honey

1. Start by peeling seasonal fruits (mangoes, peaches, bananas etc) and dice them finely.

2. Put this into a blender along with all other ingredients one by one and blend until completely smooth.

3. Strain out into a tall glass; top off with ice or frozen fruit according to your desired sweetness.

Sea Food

Eating cold water fish and other seafood offers runners almost all of their essential nutrients. In particular, seafood is packed with high energy protein as well as zinc, copper, chromium-minerals which are essential components for runners' diets. Furthermore, fish contains omega-3 fats which make it an absolute must-have in any healthy person's diet.

Studies have indicated that people who eat fish and other seafood tend to have lower risks of heart failure, vascular disease, and stroke. Eating seafood also has psychological benefits as it helps reduce depression levels.

Recent studies have demonstrated a correlation between low consumption of fish, particularly omega-3 fats, and attention deficit hyperactivity disorder (ADHD) among children. Anthropological evidence also supports this connection, showing our ancestors had higher omega-3 fatty acid intake than we currently consume today.

Fish is rich in omega-3s which have anti-inflammatory effects and may help with modern diseases like heart disease and Alzheimer's. Spicy Salmon Lettuce provides an excellent source of these healthy fats - ingredients include 5 4-ounce salmon fillets* 2 tablespoons olive oil * Lime juice * Chili Powder * Cayenne Pepper * 1 teaspoon cumin * Salt * Pepper * Head Butter lettuce, Radicchio lettuce heads and onion dices **Two tomatoes diced and 1/2 cup prepared tzatziki** Method

1. Preheat the oven or grill to 400 degrees Fahrenheit and grease a baking tray with olive oil, lime juice and spices.

3. Add the fillets to this mixture and coat them thoroughly; allow to marinate for 10 minutes.

5. Create cups of lettuce and radicchio by torning them apart with your hand, placing the radicchio cups inside lettuce ones.

6. Brush fillets with olive oil before cooking in oven or grill; cook until done.

7 Place fish fillets inside cups along with tomatoes and onions.

8. Drizzle tzatziki sauce over all before serving hot. 9. Garnish the dish by garnishing with scallions before serving hot.

Egg and Melons

Eat meat, poultry or eggs from free-range or grass-fed animals as part of a balanced diet that covers your protein needs. Add these to dairy products for quick energy boosts while providing key sources of iron and zinc (an important molecule for maintaining red blood cells), both easily absorbed through animal protein rather than other supplement sources.

Vegetarian lifestyles are equally healthy, but research suggests that a diet consisting of fruits, vegetables, whole grains and leaner cuts of meat like beef or skinless poultry may provide additional benefits by helping lower blood-cholesterol levels, maintaining blood pressure and reducing heart failure risks.

Maintaining a diet of lean proteins is paramount, so meat from animals raised on open pastures that graze on grass is preferred over stockyard-raised, corn-fed free range meat. Grass-fed animal meat tends to contain higher amounts of omega 3s and less blood vessel blocking saturated fats due to their healthier diets and higher activity levels.

This dish is one of those ideal meat dishes that won't clog your veins. * 1 chicken cut into eight pieces * 1 teaspoon ground cinnamon * Salt * Ground black pepper

5 garlic cloves minced* 2 onions chopped ** 1 1/2 tablespoons extra virgin olive oil

1/2 cup dry white wine* 1 cup chicken stock* 1 cup water

* 6 ounce can tomato paste and chopped oregano ** Method

1. Heat a pan over medium-high heat and add some sea salt, then keep aside.

2. Clean the chicken thoroughly with paper towels before drying it thoroughly.

3. In a bowl, mix together salt, cinnamon and pepper until evenly mixed.

4. Rub this mixture onto chicken pieces to coat evenly and keep aside.

5. Crush three cloves of garlic to release their flavourful oils - keep aside until use!

6. Heat a large skillet on high heat and add olive oil, then reduce heat and add chicken. Cook the chicken until brown all over (five minutes total). Take out the chicken.